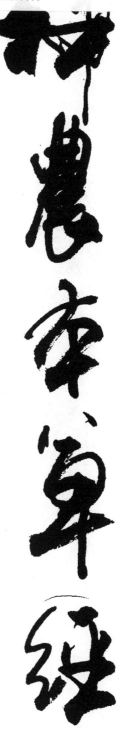

The Divine Farmer's Materia Medica

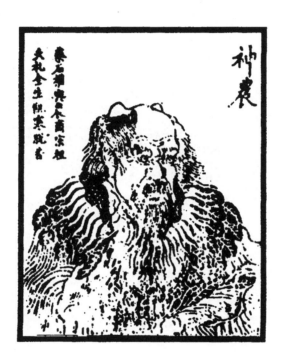

A Translation of the
Shen Nong Ben Cao Jing
by Yang Shou-zhong

BLUE POPPY PRESS, INC.
BOULDER, CO

Published by:
BLUE POPPY PRESS
A Division of Blue Poppy Enterprises, Inc.
1990 North 57th Court, Unit A
BOULDER, CO 80301

First Edition, June, 1998
Second Printing, January, 2003
Third Printing, January, 2005
Fourth Printing, October, 2005
Fifth Printing, March, 2007
Sixth Printing, October, 2007
Seventh Printing, June, 2008
Eighth Printing, April, 2009
Ninth Printing, January, 2010
Tenth Printing, November, 2010
Eleventh Printing, June, 2011
Twelfth Printing, June, 2012
Thirteenth Printing, June, 2012
Fourteenth Printing, February, 2014

ISBN 0-936185-96-1
ISBN 978-0-936185-96-5
LC 97-77991

COMP Designation: Denotative translation using a standard translational terminology

Cover caligraphy by Michael Sullivan (Seiho)

20 19 18 17 16 15 14

Printed at Edwards Brothers Malloy, Ann Arbor, MI
on recycled paper with soy inks

Publisher's Foreword

The *Shen Nong Ben Cao Jing (The Divine Farmer's Materia Medica Classic)* is one of the 10 premodern classics of Chinese medicine selected in the People's Republic of China as nationwide research priorities within the Chinese medical literature. Also referred to as the *Shen Nong Ben Jing*, the *Shen Nong Ben Cao*, the *Ben Cao Jing*, and simply the *Ben Jing*, it is one of the two most important of these 10 preeminent Chinese medical classics. The *Huang Di Nei Jing (The Yellow Emperor's Inner Classic)* is the *locus classicus* of Chinese medical theory and especially acupuncture and moxibustion, while the *Shen Nong Ben Cao Jing* is the *locus classicus* of so-called Chinese herbal medicine. All the rest of the Chinese medical literature, both premodern and contemporary, is built on the foundation of these two seminal texts. Therefore, it is not difficult to understand why we have chosen to publish this first English language translation of the *Shen Nong Ben Cao Jing* as part of Blue Poppy Press's Great Masters Series.

Shen Nong is one of the three greatest heroes of Chinese culture, the other two being the Yellow Emperor and Fu Xi, the revealer of the eight trigrams. These three legendary divine beings are credited as being the fountainhead of Chinese life-arts. The name Shen Nong can be translated as Divine Farmer, Divine Peasant, Divine Agriculturist, or Divine Husbandman. Among his numerous discoveries and revelations, Shen Nong is credited with teaching the Chinese people how to farm—thus his most common name. The first reference to a connection between Shen Nong and Chinese herbal medicine is found in the *Huai Nan Zi (The South of the Huai Master)* written by Liu An who died in 122 BCE.

> Ancient people ate grasses and drank water. They gathered the fruit from trees and ate the meat of clams. They frequently suffered from disease and poisoning. Then Shen Nong taught people for the first time how to sow the five grains, to observe whether the land was dry or wet, fertile or rocky, located in the hills or in the lowlands. He tasted the flavors of all the herbs and springs, [determining]

whether they were bitter or sweet. Thus he taught people what to avoid and where they could go. At that time, [Shen Nong] encountered 70 [herbs] in one day, [determining which were] medicines and [which were] poisons.[1]

This is the first surviving recorded instance in the Chinese literature crediting Shen Nong with determining the medicinal properties of things by tasting them himself. This story has then been repeated and embellished upon down through the centuries. Some versions even give Shen Nong a see-through stomach so he could witness the effects of what he ate on his internal organs!

The words *ben* and *cao* mean tree roots and grasses or herbs respectively. Therefore, as a compound term, they generically refer to the Chinese materia medica, and materia medica is the most commonly used translation of *ben cao* used in English today. *Ben* and *cao* are used in Chinese medicine to refer to materia medica in general because the overwhelming majority of traditional Chinese medicinals are dervied from vegetable sources. However, since the Chinese materia medica also includes mineral and animal medicinals, we have used the words, "so-called Chinese herbal medicine," above.

As mentioned previously, this work is the *locus classicus* of the *ben cao* or materia medica literature of Chinese medicine. It is this literature which describes the ingredients of Chinese medicine, their flavors and natures (*i.e.*, temperatures), their functions, and indications. According to this book, medicinals have five basic flavors—sour, salty, sweet, bitter, and acrid—and four qi or natures—cold, hot, warm, and cool. Hot diseases should be treated with cold medicinals and cold diseases should be treated with hot medicinals. This book also introduced the first method of classifying Chinese medicinals. Within this classic, all medicinals are classified into three grades or categories: superior medicinals corresponding to heaven which govern the maintenance of life and are without toxicity, medium medicinals corresponding to humankind which

---

[1] Liu An, *Huai Nan Zi*, "Xiu Wu Xun," chap. 19, p. 1a, anthologized in *Zhu Zi Ji Cheng (An Anthology of Various Masters)*, Hebei People's Press, ed. by Luan Bao-qun & Lou Xi-yuan, Tangshan, 1986.

benefit human nature and have some medicinal functions, and inferior medicinals corresponding to earth which cure disease and definitely do have some toxicity. Further, medicinals are also categorized into sovereigns, ministers, assistants, and envoys. Hence, one can find all the most basic and elemental theories of Chinese herbal medicine in seminal form in this classic.

Although a book titled the Shen Nong Jing (The Divine Farmer's Classic) is mentioned by various Chinese medical authors and Daoists interested in longevity practices in the Qin dynasty (221-206 BCE), this book has long been lost, and it is not at all clear that it was, in fact, an early version of this materia medica. The first mention of the Shen Nong Ben Cao per se is found in the writings of the Daoist physician Tao Hong-jing whom lived from 452-536 CE. According to Tao, the knowledge of Chinese materia medica transmitted orally from the time of Shen Nong was first written down in the later Han dynasty (circa 200 CE). As Paul U. Unschuld says in his Medicine in China: A History of Pharmaceutics, "This opinion was based upon the fact that the names used for the places of origin of the drugs in the various pen-ts'ao works of T'ao's time were common to the later Han period."[2]

In fact, it is due to the writings of Tao Hong-jing that we have any version of the Shen Nong Ben Cao Jing today. Tao is the author of the Ben Cao Jing Ji Zhu (Collected Annotations on the Materia Medica Classic) and a Shen Nong Ben Cao Jing. According to Unschuld, these are the same book and sometimes they are referred to jointly as the Shen Nong Ben Cao Jing Ji Zhu. Tao wrote the Shen Nong Ben Cao Jing first in three books and later revised this into the Ben Cao Jing Ji Zhu in seven books based on Daoist cosmological beliefs involving the number seven. However, the contents of these two books are identical. In his preface, Tao mentions three main sources for his work. These include several different versions of the Shen Nong Ben Cao Jing, the Tong Jun Cai Yao Lu (Gentleman Tong's Notes on Gathering Medicinals), and the Lei Kung Yao Dui (Lei Kung's Comparison of Medicinals). He also mentions Zhang Chi (142-220? CE), Hua Tuo (190-265 CE), and Hua Tuo's students, Wu Pu and Li Dang-zhi, as authors before

---

[2]   Unschuld, Paul U., Medicine in China: A History of Pharmaceutics, U. of CA Press, Berkeley, 1986, p. 17

him who had worked on earlier versions of the *Shen Nong Ben Cao Jing.* However, as Unschuld states, "It can no longer be proved whether there was, in fact, ever a specific, original work entitled *Shen-nung pen-ts'ao ching,* or whether various pharmaceutical collections of the Han period were written with this or a similar title."[3]

In any case, even Tao Hong-jing's *Shen Nong Ben Cao Jing* and *Ben Cao Jing Ji Zhu* were lost. Nevertheless, efforts to recreate the *Shen Nong Ben Cao Jing* were undertaken at least as early as the Song dynasty (960-1280 CE). This may sound crazy to Western readers not familiar with premodern Chinese literary practices. If something is lost, it's lost. However, it was not uncommon for Chinese authors to include whole books or at least chapters from previous books into their own new compilations. This was an accepted literary practice and carried no opprobium of plagiarism as it would in the contemporary West. This process was made easier by the fact that Tao Hong-jing had used two different colors of ink in his version of the *Shen Nong Ben Cao Jing.* Everything written in red ink was supposed to be the words of Shen Nong. Since succeeding authors of later *ben cao* continued this convention, it makes the identification of quotes from the *Shen Nong Ben Cao Jing* somewhat easier.

As early as the Tang dynasty (618-907 CE), Sun Si-miao had incorporated lengthy sections of the *Shen Nong Ben Cao Jing* into his own *Qian Jin Fang (Prescriptions [Worth] a Thousand [Pieces of] Gold),* and this book has survived until today. It is one of the earliest sources for recompiling the *Shen Nong Ben Cao Jing.* The *Jing Shi Zheng Lei Bei Ji Ben Cao (A Classic & Historic [Work]: A Materia Medica for Emergencies [Based on] Pattern Categorization)* compiled by Tang Shen-wei in 1108 CE is the most important surviving source for recreating the *Shen Nong Ben Cao Jing.* However, even Li Shi-zhen's late Ming dynasty (1368-1644 CE) *Ben Cao Gang Mu (Great Outline of Materia Medica)* has been used to help recreate this seminal materia medica classic, since even Li maintained the convention of using red and black inks in order to identify the supposed words of the divine Shen Nong.

---

[3] *Ibid.,* p. 17

At this point, the reader should remember that in ancient times, doctors would copy other doctor's copies of books by hand. Therefore, different copyists often took the liberty of rearranging texts depending on their own tastes and proclivities, just as modern college students might rearrange their teacher's lecture notes in order to facilitate their own study. Because of this, several different versions of the *Zheng Lei Ben Cao* currently exist, and, therefore, there are a number of different versions of the *Shen Nong Ben Cao* available today. The main discrepancies between these existing versions of the *Shen Nong Ben Cao* are 1) the number of medicinals they include, 2) the format of their presentation, and 3) the texts on certain particular medicinals. It is believed that the original *Ben Cao Jing* contained 365 medicinals. However, all extant versions fall short of this number despite many previous scholars' efforts to recover these lost medicinals. In terms of format, some versions have four books, while others have only three. Some versions simply divide all the medicinals into superior, medium, and inferior grades, while others first divide them into wood, grass, animal, and stone medicinals which are then subdivided into superior, medium, and inferior grades. Some versions contain a table of contents at their beginning and others do not. Still others give a list of medicinals to be discussed before each section of each book. In addition, there are minor discrepancies in the text itself under each medicinal. For instance, some versions discuss the geographic origins of the medicinals, while others do not. This last discrepancy is based on the assumption by certain editors that this information was a later addition and not part of the original text.

The present translation is based on the *Ben Cao Jing (Materia Medica Classic)* edited by Cao Yuan-yu and published by the Shanghai Science & Technology Press in Shanghai in 1987. It is Yang Shou-zhong's opinion that this version is the most carefully collated and edited of the various versions available in the People's Republic of China and is probably closer to the original than any other. The most popular current version of this seminal medicinal classic is the *Shen Nong Ben Cao Jing (The Divine Farmer's Materia Medica Classic)* published by the Chinese Medical Classics Publishing House in Beijing in 1982. Readers familiar with that version should note that these two are not the same. The present version differs from the *Ben Cao Jing* version in that it includes a Book Four. This is comprised of those passages which are absent from our source text but which are common to many other versions. Specifically, these are segments included as appendices at the end of the *Shen Nong Ben Cao Jing* edited by Huang Shi. Huang Shi was a high-ranking official during the reigns of Jia Qing (1796-1820 CE) and Dao Guang (1821-1850 CE). In addition, we have created a new Table of Contents to make this book easier to use for modern readers and we have deleted the listing of medicinals discussed in each chapter as superfluous given the Table of Contents and index of medicinals at the back. Insertions within brackets have been added by the translator in order to bring out the meaning of the text and render it in better English while allowing readers to identify the words which actually are in the source text.

The terminology and methodology used in this translation is based on Nigel Wiseman and Ken Boss's *Glossary of Chinese Medical Terms and Acupuncture Points*, Paradigm Publications, Brookline, MA, 1990, with updates and revisions as contained in Nigel Wiseman's *English-Chinese Chinese-English Dictionary of Chinese Medicine*, Hunan Science & Technology Press, Changsha, 1995. The medicinals are identified by their Chinese names written in Pinyin followed by their Latinate pharmacological nomenclature in parentheses. Sources for these Latinate identifications are Bensky and Gamble's *Chinese Herbal Medicine: Materia Medica, Revised Edition*, Eastland Press, Seattle, 1993; Hong-yen Hsu's *Oriental Materia Medica: A Concise Guide*, Oriental Healing Arts Institute, Long Beach, CA, 1986; Stuart and Read's *Chinese Materia Medica*, Southern Materials Center, Taipei, 1979; Paul U. Unschuld's *Medicine in China: A History of Pharmaceutics*, U. of CA Press, Berkeley, 1986; *A Barefoot Doctor's Manual, Revised & Enlarged Edition*, Cloudburst Press, Mayne Isle, WA, 1977; and the *Zhong Yao Da Ci Dian (Large Dictionary of Chinese Medicinals)*, Shanghai Science & Technology Press, Shanghai, 1991. In particular, Stuart & Read's *Chinese Materia Medica* is a good resource for finding the Chinese characters for the medicinals in this text as well as discussions of their botanical identifications and common English names. When a medicinal is subsequently discussed in a footnote, we have simply referred to it by its capitalized common English name or a simplified version of its Latin botanical name in nominative case. Regrettably, the translator was unable to find Latin (or English) identifications for a very small handful of medicinals. Hopefully, as scholars in China continue to research this classic, these will be added to future editions of this work.

Westerns often think of Chinese medicine as Daoist medicine. In most cases, this is a benign myth. In actual fact, the overwhelming majority of the great books of Chinese medicine were written by authors who identified themselves as Confucianist. However, the *Shen Nong Ben Cao Jing* is definitely an example of the Daoist contribution to the development of Chinese medicine. As the reader will see, there is a great interest on the part of the author in using so-called herbs in order to achieve immortality and other supernatural powers and abilities. In addition, there are more references to demonology in this book than to the essentially Confucian medicine of systematic correspondences. Modern readers coming across references to flying in the sky and warding off demons and ghosts through the administration of Chinese medicinals should understand the historical context and provenance of this seminal classic *and take the information with a large grain of salt!* It should also be remembered that many Chinese, including emperors and even famous doctors such as Huang-fu Mi, made themselves ill and even cut off their lives prematurely by taking such external elixirs compounded out of potentially toxic materials.

Nevertheless, when it comes to Chinese materia medica, the two great books are the *Shen Nong Ben Cao Jing* (contained herein) and Li Shi-zhen's *Ben Cao Gang Mu (Great Outline of Materia Medica)*. It is with great pleasure that Blue Poppy Press is able to make this first English language translation of the *Shen Nong Ben Cao Jing* available to Western scholars and practitioners of Chinese medicine as part of our Great Masters Series. Hopefully this translation will help deepen the Western understanding of the history and development of Chinese herbal medicine. In particular, we believe it will be useful for professional practitioners to compare these early Chinese medicinal descriptions with standard contemporary descriptions as found in Bensky and Gamble's *Chinese Herbal Medicine: Materia Medica*. Such a comparison will afford a better understanding of the evolution of contemporary Chinese medicine at least in terms of materia medica. For more information on the history and development of the *ben cao* literature in China, the reader is referred to Paul U. Unschuld's excellent *Medicine in China: A History of Pharmaceutics*.

Bob Flaws
Boulder, CO

Book One

Preface to the *Ben Cao Jing*

There are 120 superior class medicinals which are used as sovereigns.[4] They mainly nourish life and correspond to heaven. They are nontoxic and taking them in large amounts and for a long time will not harm people. If one intends to make one's body light,[5] boost the qi, prevent

---

[4] Superior class medicinals are superior in a number of different ways. In brief, they are nontoxic medicinals that are able to nurture life and therefore bestow longevity. In contrast, medium grade or middle class medicinals are able to cultivate personality or modify temperament, as are, for example, *He Huan* (Cortex Albizziae Julibrissinis) and *Xuan Cao* (Radix Hemerocallis Fulvae). The former resolves anger, while the latter is able to help relieve worry. Since this class of medicinals may be toxic, their prescription requires care. Inferior class medicinals specifically treat disease. They are usually at least slightly toxic. This means that they cannot be taken in large amounts or for prolonged periods of time without developing negative side effects. In our source text, there are 119 superior class medicinals, 120 middle class medicinals, and 122 inferior class medicinals. Put together, there are 361 medicinals, four short of 365.

The terms sovereign, minister, and envoy and assistant in this text do not mean what they have now come to mean in Chinese medicine. In this case, they are simply synonyms of superior, middle and inferior class medicinals. Later medical thinkers enlarged on these terms and now the principal ingredient in a formula is the sovereign, while the other components are ministers, assistants, and envoys.

[5] This implies not only limberness but also the acquisition of such supernormal abilities as the power to fly or to walk a thousand *li* without becoming tired. Such references underscore that it was principally the Daoists who created the early materia medica literature. In that case, they were not primarily concerned with the treatment of disease but the achievement of "immortality" and various extraordinary powers through the ingestion of various "elixirs."

aging,[6] and prolong life, one should base [one's efforts] on the superior class.[7]

There are 120 medium class medicinals which are used as ministers.[4] They mainly nurture personality[8] and correspond to humanity. They may or may not be toxic, and [therefore,] one should weigh and ponder before putting them to their appropriate use. If one intends to control disease, supplement vacuity, and replenish exhaustion, one should base [one's efforts] on the middle class.[9]

There are 125 inferior class medicinals which are used as assistants and envoys.[4] They mainly treat disease and correspond to earth. They are usually toxic and cannot be taken for a long time. If one intends to eliminate cold and heat and evil qi,[10] break accumulations and gatherings, and cure disease, one should base [one's efforts] on the inferior class.[9]

Medicinals [in a prescription] are classified as the sovereign, minister, assistant, and envoy. To achieve synergism and coordination, it is

---

[6]   The Chinese literally says "no aging." This again belies the Daoist preoccupation with elixirs of immortality conferring extreme longevity. It does not just mean the slowing of the aging process and prevention of untimely senility.

[7]   This passage corresponds to the initial section of Book Four. It has been purposefully preserved for readers to make a comparison between different versions.

[8]   It was believed that some medicinals are effective for treating disease and, at the same time, are good for the cultivation of various virtues in human beings.

[9]   The second and the third passage combined correspond to the second passage in our Book Four. See note 4 above. In many other versions, there is no phrase corresponding to the part from "one should base" to the end of the sentence. In that case, the sentence can be rendered as: "[The medicinals] are intended to make the body light...or control disease..."

[10]   Here, evil qi refers to sudden, serious conditions and/or mental-neurological problems, such as epilepsy, pestilential wind, and malign stroke. The latter is a sudden loss of consciousness or sudden contraction of paralysis. In sometimes later sections this term means no more than a sudden, serious condition.

appropriate to use one sovereign, two ministers, and five assistants. It is also possible to use one sovereign, three ministers, and nine assistants and envoys.[11]

Medicinals should coordinate [with each other] in terms of yin and yang, like mother and child or brothers.[12] They may be roots, stalks, flowers, or fruits [of a plant], and they may be herbs, stones, bones, or flesh. Some [medicinals] can go [i.e., be used] alone. Some need each other. Some mutually reinforce [each other]. Some fear each other. Some are averse to each other. Some clash with each other. Some kill each other. These seven emotions [i.e., relationships] require that, when combining [medicinals], it is proper to use those that need each other and are mutually empowering. One should not use those that are mutually averse or mutually clash. As

---

[11]   This refers to the proportions of the amounts of ingredients in a formula. One sovereign and two ministers is called an odd prescription. It is for so-called near disease. One sovereign and three ministers is an even prescription. It is designed for so-called distant disease. On the one hand, a sovereign medicinal is one from the superior class. On the other hand, it also may refer to the main ingredient in a formula which has a direct action on the disease. Minister, assistant, and envoy medicials should be understood in a similar way.

[12]   Medicinals are divided into yin and yang depending on their natures and actions. Those that are ascending and effusing are yang, while those that provoke vomiting or are precipitating are yin. Those which are acrid, sweet, and heat-generating are yang, and those that are bitter, sour, and salty are yin. Those which are rich in flavor are yang, while those with a bland flavor are yin. Medicinals that tranquilize and are sluggish in action are yin. In contrast, those that easily and quickly penetrate are yang. Those which are able to move the qi division are yang, while those able to move the blood division are yin.

As to mother and child, etc., there are two different interpretations. According to one interpretation, the various medicinals in a prescription should work in a well coordinated way similar to a mother and her child or between brothers. According to another interpretation, various medicinals in a formula should have a five phase relationship between the generator and the generated (mother and child) and between assistants or envoys (brothers). However, this latter interpretation is controversial. In fact, there is a conspicuous lack of five phase systematic correspondence theory in this text. Unschuld explains this in terms of the Daoist proclivities of the early ben cao authors who rejected the model of systematic correspondence along with other Confucian-Legalist notions.

for toxic medicinals, they should be processed with those to which they are averse or with those that kill them. Otherwise they cannot be used in combination.

Medicinals may have five flavors—sour, salty, sweet, bitter, and acrid. Furthermore, they have four qi—cold, hot, warm, and cool.[13] They may be toxic or nontoxic. Whether they should be dried in the shade or in the sun, which seasons and months they should be collected and processed in, whether they should be used raw or after processing, where they should be produced, whether they are genuine or fake, or old or new, all this has a method to go by.

Because of their natures, some medicinals are appropriate for pills, others for powders, some for boiling in water, others for soaking in wine, and [yet] others for boiling down to a paste. There are also cases where one material is suitable for various forms. Some, [however,] cannot be put in water or wine. One should follow the natures of medicinals and must not violate these.

In order to treat a disease, one should first make a study of its origin and observe its mechanisms. Before the five viscera become vacuous, the six bowels are exhausted, the blood vessels [i.e., the pulse] become chaotic,[14] and the essence spirit is dissipated, administration of medicinals will surely result in survival. If disease has already taken shape, then half recovery can be achieved. If the disease condition has gone too far, it will be hard to restore the life.

When treating disease with toxic medicinals, one should first use a sorghum grain-sized amount. Once the disease is gone, one should stop

[13] Nowhere subsequently in the body of this classic are the four qi or natures mentioned. Only flavor is attributed under each medicinal's individual discussion. The concept of the four qi as part of a medicinal's nature was a later advance in Chinese medical theory. Therefore, this section must have been added by some later editor.

[14] The term chaotic pulse should be understood in a general way. It does not merely mean a terribly arrhythmic pulse. A pulse which is incongruous with the season or the disease is also called a chaotic pulse.

using it. If the disease is yet to leave, double the amount. If it is still there, increase the amount 10 times. The amount is measured by the removal of the disease.

To treat cold, one should use hot medicinals. To treat heat, one should use cold medicinals. For nondispersion of drink and food, one should prescribe ejecting and precipitating medicinals. For demonic influx and *gu* toxins,[15] one should prescribe toxic medicinals. For welling abscesses and swellings, sores and tumors, one should prescribe wound medicinals.[16] For

---

[15] The terms demonic influx (*gui zhu*) and *gu* toxins (*gu du*) are often mentioned in juxtaposition as a single concept. Demonic influx is a synonym of cadaverous influx (*shi zhu*). The word demonic (*gui*) can be defined as terrible, intractable, or fatal, while influx (*zhu*) means infectiousness. Therefore, demonic influx usually refers to an infectious disease of sudden onset manifesting acute abdominal pain, cold and heat, masses in the rib-side region, and aching pain everywhere in the body which baffles location. This disease may last years before it finally ends in death. In some contexts, demonic influx may also refer to *lao zhai* (taxation consumption) or tuberculosis in modern terms.

Gu toxins refer to disease caused by imaginary or real poisonous worms. These were believed to cause unbearable stomachache, fulminant swelling, blood ejection, and derangement. In premodern texts, many disorders with unclear causes are often spoken of as *gu* toxins. Sun Si-miao (581-682 CE) said:

There are a thousand kinds of *gu* toxins which differ from each other. These may manifest as precipitating fresh blood; a desire to stay in a dark room, hating light; a perverse mood, now being angry but now happy; or heaviness of the limbs with aching and soreness in the hundreds of joints. There is no end to their manifestations. Some cases will not die until three years after contraction. Some acute cases die in a month or 100 days. On death, [the worms] never fail to exit from the nine portals or through the rib-side.

[16] Wound medicinals are those that disperse binding (*i.e.*, scatter nodulation), free the flow of the channels, disinhibit the orifices, dispel wind, transform phlegm, and precipitate blood stasis. In addition, such medicinals are often applied externally.

xiii

wind dampness, one should prescribe wind dampness medicinals.[17] In all [cases], one should follow appropriately [*i.e.*, match the medicinals to the nature of the disease].

If the disease is located above the diaphragm in the chest, one should take the medicinals after meals. If the disease is located below the heart [or] in the abdomen, one should take the medicinals before meals. If the disease is located in the four limbs or the blood vessels, it is proper to take the medicinals on an empty stomach in the morning. If the disease is located in the bones and marrow, it is proper to take the medicinals on a full stomach in the evening.

---

[17] E.g., *Fang Feng* (Radix Ledebouriellae Divaricatae), *Bai Zhu* (Rhixoma Atractylodis Macrocephalae), *Chai Hu* (Radix Bupleuri), and *Gui Zhi* (Ramulus Cinnamomi Cassiae)

The great diseases mainly include wind stroke, cold damage,[18] cold and heat,[19] warm malaria,[20] malign stroke,[21] sudden turmoil,[22] enlarged abdomen, water swelling, intestinal afflux[23] and dysentery, inhibited urination and defecation, running piglet,[24] qi ascent, cough and counterflow,[25] retching and vomiting, jaundice, wasting thirst, lodged

---

[18] Wind stroke and cold damage here imply two patterns of cold damage disease. When wind cold strikes a person, it gives rise to the illness of cold damage. If it manifests spontaneous sweating and a moderate pulse, it is known as wind stroke. If it is characterized by absence of perspiration and a tight pulse, it is called cold damage.

[19] Cold and heat may refer to alternating fever and chills, but more often they refer to fever with aversion to cold.

[20] Warm malaria is a specific type of malaria in which the attack of fever precedes the chills or fever is followed by an absence of chills.

[21] Malign stroke is similar to demonic influx and *gu* toxins. Sometimes these are difficult to distinguish. It covers a large spectrum of variegated diseases or problems. There are 14 species of malign stroke which even include committing suicide by hanging, drowning, summerheat stroke, and frostbite. According to the *Zhu Bing Yuan Hou Lun (Origins & Symptoms of Various Diseases)* published by Chao Yuan-fang in 610 CE, malign stroke "is stroke by a demonic or spiritual qi under the condition of debilitated essence and spirit." Its main signs and symptoms are sudden onset, cold and heat, heart and abdominal pain, generalized pain, blood ejection and hemafecia, inhibited breathing, urinary and fecal stoppage, and arched-back rigidity.

[22] Sudden turmoil is a result of the mutual interference between the clear and turbid qi. Its manifetations are mainly sudden onset with simultaneous vomiting and diarrhea.

[23] Intestinal afflux refers to dysentery with hemafecia.

[24] Running piglet is also called kidney accumulation. It refers to qi starting from the lower abdomen and rushing to the heart. This qi often moves up and down irregularly.

[25] Qi ascent is a trouble accompanying coughing, similar to asthma in modern terms. Qi ascent and counterflow cough are often mentioned as one single trouble. Then its translation is cough with counterflow qi ascent.

rheum and food aggregation,[26] hardness and accumulation, concretions and conglomerations,[27] fright evil,[28] withdrawal and epilepsy, demonic influx, throat impediment,[29] toothache, deafness, blindness, incised wounds, broken bones, welling abscesses and swellings, malign sores, hemorrhoids and fistulas, and goiters and tumors. In males, there are five taxations and seven damages,[30] vacuity and fatigue, languor and emaciation, while in females, there are vaginal discharge, flooding, and blood block. [Besides,] there are wounds caused by worm and snakebite and damage done by *gu* toxins. The above is a [short] synopsis.

One should base [the treatment of disease] on its primary [pattern] which may [then] have variants. [These variants] can be likened to branches and leaves.[31] [Then] it is proper to make a prescription in accordance with the signs they show.

---

[26] Lodged rheum and food aggregation constitute a syndrome which centers around indigestion. Its manifestations may include chest fullness and glomus, emaciation, alternating cold and heat, no appetite, and abnormal defecation.

[27] Hardness and accumulation mean accumulation and gathering which in turn can be synonymous with concretions and conglomerations. A concretion is a tangible mass which is fixed in location, while a conglomeration is an intangible mass which comes and goes and may move about.

[28] This term is synonymous with fright wind as usually seen in children.

[29] Throat impediment often does not simply mean sore throat. It is characterized by sore throat, difficulty swallowing and speaking, and sometimes dryness in the mouth, vexation, and a curled tongue.

[30] The five taxations refers to taxations of the five viscera. This term is derived from the *Nei Jing (Inner Classic)*, which says, "Protracted looking damages the blood [*i.e.*, the heart]; protracted lying damages the qi [*i.e.*, the lungs]..." However, this term may also refer to affect taxation, thought taxation, heart taxation, worry taxation, and emaciation taxation. The seven damages or injuries are liver damage, heart damage, spleen damage, lung damage, kidney damage, bone damage, and vessel damage.

[31] This sentence implies that a pattern may have several variants or sub-patterns. The primary pattern is the root, while its variants or sub-patterns are the branches and leaves growing out of it.

Table of Contents

Ben Cao Jing
Book Two

Jades and Stones: Superior Class

Yu Quan **(Nephritum)** is sweet and balanced.[32] It mainly treats hundreds of diseases of the five viscera. It limbers the sinews and strengthens the bones, quiets the ethereal and corporeal souls, promotes the growth of the muscles and flesh, and boosts the qi. Protracted taking may cultivate endurance to cold and summerheat and make one free from hunger and thirst[33] to become a non-aging immortal. If one takes five catties [*i.e.*, 500g

---

[32]   *Yu Quan* literally means jade spring. There is reason to suspect that this is a typographical error and that this should read *Yu Xue* (Jade Dust). It is said that, in olden times, there was the practice of grinding Jade into powder and then taking it to keep fit and prevent disease.

Usually, the character of a medicinal is mainly described in terms of its flavor and its qi (*i.e.*, temperature or nature). The five flavors are sweet, bitter, acrid, sour, and salty, while the four qi include cold, hot, warm, and cool. Medicinals that are neither cold or hot, neither warm or cool are called level or balanced. Take Talcum for example. Its flavor is sweet, while its qi is cold. However, at the time this work was written, a medicinal's flavor and qi were not distinguished. Rather, these two were incorporated into one single concept—flavor. Therefore, a typical medicinal description in our source text might read that it has a sweet and cold flavor. Because this sounds quite curious in English, we have simply omitted the word flavor altogether.

[33]   It is said that if one has reached a certain level in the *Dao* through self-cultivation or by taking certain medicinals, one may live for long periods of time without eating and drinking without suffering any deleterious effect. In Asia, this belief is common to Daoism, Buddhism, Hinduism, and Jainism.

of it] when dying, one's complexion will remain unchanged for three years after death. Its other name is *Yu Zha* (Jade Sweet Wine).

Dan Sha (Cinnabar)[34] is sweet and slightly cold. It treats hundreds of diseases of the five viscera and the body. It nurtures the essence spirit, quiets the ethereal and corporeal souls, boosts the qi, brightens the eyes, and kills spirit demons and evil malign ghosts.[35] Protracted taking may enable one to communicate with the spirit light[36] and prevent senility. It is capable of transforming into mercury. It is produced in mountains and valleys [or mountain valleys].

Shui Yin (Mercurius) is acrid and cold. It mainly treats scabs, itching sores, and bald white scalp sores, kills worms and lice on the skin, induces abortion, and eliminates fever. It kills the toxins of gold, silver, copper, and tin. When melted, it reduces to Cinnabar. Protracted taking may make one an ever-living immortal. It is produced from the earth in the plains.

---

[34] Cinnabar is now mainly used to treat confused spirit, fright palpitations, fearful throbbing, and insomnia. However, because it is also able to boost the blood and the qi, it is often prescribed to supplement blood and qi vacuity in order to quiet the spirit. Because it is a heavy medicinal, tending to downbear, it can also be used to suppress retching and vomiting.

[35] Demonology was one of three models of disease current in China when this book was originally compiled in the late Han dynasty. This is reflected in numerous mentions to demons and ghosts in this text. The other two medical models current in China during this period were magical correspondence and systematic correspondence. Because of the Daoist provenance of this text, systematic correspondence is largely lacking herein and, where it does appear, may be a later interpolation. Affliction by demons and ghosts causes such disorders as palpitations, fearful throbbing, and clouded spirit or, in modern terms, mental-emotional derangement.

[36] Communication with the spirit light is another supernatural ability sought for by Daoist adepts through self-cultivation and the ingestion of elixirs. It refers to supernatural vision as in seeing the past or future or seeing events occuring at a distance.

2

Kong Qing (**Azuritum**)[37] is sweet and cold. It mainly treats clear-eye blindness and deafness, brightens the eyes, disinhibits the nine orifices, frees the flow of the blood vessels, and nurtures the essence spirit. Protracted taking may make the body light, prolong life, and prevent senility. It is able to transform copper, iron, lead, and tin into gold. It is produced in mountains and valleys.

Ceng Qing (**Azuritum**) is sour and a little cold. It mainly treats eye pain, relieves tearing and wind impediment,[38] disinhibits the joints, frees the nine orifices, and breaks concretions and conglomerations, accumulations and gatherings. Protracted taking may make the body light and prevent senility. It is able to transform into gold and copper. It is produced in mountains and valleys.

Bai Qing (**Azuritum**) is sweet and balanced. It mainly brightens the eyes, disinhibits the nine orifices, [treats] deafness and evil qi below the heart, provokes vomiting in people, and kills various toxins and the three [kinds of] worms.[39] Protracted taking may enable one to communicate with the spirit light, make the body light, prolong life, and prevent senility. It is produced in mountains and valleys.

---

[37] This medicinal and the next three are all derived from the same mineral source. They all exist in nature in the form of ore. However, this ore may be found in different shapes and, hence, the three different ingredients. *Kong Qing* is a round shape with a hollow center. *Ceng Qing* is found in stratified layers. *Bian Qing* is found in short cylinders. *Bai Qing* is the same substance as *Bian Qing* but is white.

[38] Wind impediment refers to migratory joint pain due to wind, cold, and dampness with wind as the prevalent factor. It is usually accompanied by aching pain in the flesh.

[39] This refers to the various kinds of parasites within the body. Chao Yuan-fang (5th-6th centuries CE), the author of the *Zhu Bing Yuan Hou Lun* (*Treatise on the Origins & Symptoms of Various Diseases*), says that the three worms are pinworms, roundworms, and red worms. Red worms are described as a flesh-colored worm causing rumbling intestines, abdominal pain, diarrhea, and, occasionally, hemafecia.

Bian Qing (**Azuritum**) is a little cold and nontoxic. It mainly treats eye pain, brightens the eyes, and [heals] fracture [caused by] falls as well as welling abscesses and swellings, and refractory incised wounds. It breaks accumulations and gatherings, resolves toxic qi, and disinhibits the essence spirit. Protracted taking may make the body light and prevent senility. It is produced in mountains and valleys.

Yun Mu (**Muscovitum**) is sweet and balanced. It mainly treats dead muscles and skin in the body[40] as well as wind stroke cold and heat [with dizziness and sickness] as if on board a cart or boat. It eliminates evil qi, quiets the five viscera, boosts the fetal essence [*i.e.*, semen], brightens the eyes, makes the body light, and prolongs life. Its other name is *Yun Hua* (Cloud Flower). Yet another name is *Yun Ying* (Cloud Floret). It is also called *Yun Ye* (Cloud Fluid), *Yun Sha* (Cloud Sand), and *Lin Shi* (Fluorescent Stone). It is produced in mountains and valleys.

Po Xiao (**Slaked Lime**) is bitter and cold. It is nontoxic and mainly treats hundreds of diseases. It eliminates cold and heat and evil qi and expels accumulations and gatherings in the six bowels as well as firmly bound retention and aggregation [of water and food]. It is able to transform 72 kinds of stone. If it is taken after being sublimated, it may make one an immortal with a light body. It is produced in mountains and valleys.

Xiao Shi (**Mirabilitum**)[41] is bitter and cold. It mainly treats accumulated heat in the five viscera and stomach distention and block. It flushes away accumulated abiding drink and food, weeds out the old to bring forth the new, and eliminates evil qi. It may be sublimated into a paste. Protracted taking may make the body light. It is also named *Mang Xiao* (Aristate Lime). It is produced in mountains and valleys.

---

[40] Dead muscles refer to a sensation of itching in the flesh like wriggling worms, *i.e.*, formication.

[41] Mirabilitum is a very good cathartic which is often prescribed to precipitate or purge food and drink accumulation from the stomach and intestines. However, in this text, the translator suspects that Mirabilitum and Slaked Lime have been mistakenly juxtaposed in terms of their indications.

4

Fan Shi **(Alumen)** is sour and cold. It mainly treats cold and heat, diarrhea and dysentery, white ooze [*i.e.*, white vaginal discharge], genital erosion, malign sores, and eye pain. It fortifies the bones and teeth. If it is taken after being sublimated, it may make the body light, prevent senility, and lengthen life. It is also named *Yu Nie* (Feather Alumen). It is produced in mountains and valleys.

Hua Shi **(Talcum)**[42] is sweet and cold. It mainly treats generalized fever, afflux diarrhea, difficult lactation in women, and dribbling urinary block. It disinhibits urination, flushes accumulations and gatherings in the stomach [with] cold and heat, and boosts the essential qi. Protracted taking may make the body light and free from hunger and it may prolong life. It is produced in the mountains and valleys in Zhe Yang.[43]

Zi Shi **(Flouritum)** is sweet and balanced. It mainly treats the heart and abdomen, cough and counterflow, and evil qi. It supplements insufficiency and [hence treats] women with 10 year old infertility due to cold wind in the child's palace [*i.e.*, uterus]. Protracted taking may make the center warm, the body light, and prolong life. It is produced in the valleys of Mount Tai.[44]

Bai Shi Ying **(Quartz Crystal)** is sweet and slightly warm. It mainly treats wasting thirst, impotence, yin [essence] insufficiency, cough and counterflow, and enduring cold in the chest around the diaphragm. It boosts the qi and eliminates wind damp impediment. Protracted taking may make the body light and lengthen life. It is produced in mountains and valleys.

---

[42] Talcum is also able to clear summerheat and both internal and external heat, quench vexatious thirst, and cure fulminant diarrhea, dysentery with pressure on the rectum, and vaginal discharge.

[43] This was an ancient county in the precincts of present-day Shandong Province.

[44] This refers to the mountains in what is now Shandong Province.

Qing Shi, Chi Shi, Huang Shi, Bai Shi, Hei Shi (Halloysitum Viridis, Rubrum, Aureum, Album, Negrum, etc.)[45] are sweet and balanced. They mainly treat jaundice, diarrhea and dysentery, intestinal afflux with pus and blood, genital erosion, precipitation of blood, red and white [vaginal discharge], evil qi, welling abscesses and swellings, flat abscesses, hemorrhoids, malign sores, head sores, and itching scabs. Protracted taking may replenish the marrow, boost the qi, and make one fat and strong, free from hunger, and the body light while prolonging life. The five colors of Halloysitum [each] respectively supplement the five viscera in accordance with their colors.[46]

Tai Yi Yu Yu Liang (Limonitum)[47] is sweet and balanced. It mainly treats cough and counterflow qi ascent, concretions and conglomerations, blood block, and leaking. It eliminates evil qi. Protracted taking may build endurance to cold or summerheat and hunger and make one an immortal with a body so light as to be able to fly a thousand *li*. Its other name is *Shi Nao* (Stone Brain). It is produced in mountains and valleys.

Yu Yu Liang (Limonitum) is sweet and cold. It mainly treats cough and counterflow, cold and heat, vexatious fullness, red and white dysentery, blood block, concretions and conglomerations, and great fever. Taking it

---

[45] The identities of these medicinals are controversial. Many people believe that all except for *Hei Shi Zhi* are variously colored Kaolinite clays, while *Hei Shi Zhi* is a kind of Graphite.

[46] The five viscera correspond respectively to the five colors: the heart to red, the lungs to white, the liver to green-blue, the spleen to yellow, and the kidneys to black. It follows then that, for example, Halloysitum Album supplements the lungs, while Hallyositum Rubrum supplements the heart, etc.

[47] *Tai Yi Yu Yu Liang* can be literally translated as the Surplus Provisions of Yu of Great Supremacy. Great Supremacy (*Tai Yi*) was the teacher of legendary Yu who was the founder of China's first empire. Therefore, this medicinal was regarded as a divine medicinal. Actually, however, it is the same substance as the next one (*Yu Yu Liang*). In ancient times, two forms of this single substance were identified based on their different areas of production.

after it is sublimated may make one free from hunger, the body light, and prolong life. It is produced in pools and swamps.[48]

Xiong Huang (Realgar) is bitter and balanced. It mainly treats cold and heat, mouse fistulas,[49] malign sores, flat abscesses, hemorrhoids, and dead muscles. It kills spiritual matters,[50] vicious demons, evil qi, and hundreds of toxic worms and insects. It overpowers the five weapons.[51] Taking it after it is sublimated may make one an immortal with a light body. Its other name is *Huang Shi Shi* (Yellow Edible Stone). It is produced in mountains and valleys.

---

[48] In ancient times, *Tai Yi Yu Yu Liang* and *Yu Yu Liang* were differentiated according to their different places of production. That produced in the mountains was referred to as *Tai Yi Yu Yu Liang*, while plain *Yu Yu Liang* was believed to be formed under water.

In most but not all cases throughout this work where a medicinal is said to grow or be produced in the pool or in the river, the real meaning is that the medicinal is a lowland product found near water rather than an aquatic product per se.

[49] *I.e.*, tubercular lymphadenopathy in the neck and the armpit

[50] Spiritual matter simply means a spirit or ghost which causes a sudden, fulminant disease usually accompanied by mental disorders such as delirious speech and hallucinations. In ancient times, it was believed that there was a spirit which resided inside every animate or inanimate thing and that this spirit might act in the world at large in either a benevolent or malevolent way. In particular, weasels and foxes were believed to be possessed by malevolent spirits which might negatively afflict human beings.

[51] The five weapons refer to commonly used weapons in premodern times, for example, the spear and pike. This sentence implies that Realgar possesses a supernatural protective power when worn as an amulet. Carrying it on one's body was believed to make a warrior invulnerable in battle.

7

Jades and Stones: Middle Class

Shi Dan (**Cuprus Sulphate**)[52] is sour and a little cold. It mainly brightens the eyes [and treats] eye pain, incised wounds, and all [kinds of] epilepsy and tetany. [It treats] genital erosion and pain in females, stone strangury, cold and heat, flooding and precipitation of blood, and various kinds of evil and toxic qi. It makes pregnancy possible. Taking it after it is sublimated may prevent senility, while protrated taking may increase longevity and make one an immortal. It may change iron into copper, gold, or silver. Its other name is *Bi Shi* (Green Stone). It is produced in mountains and valleys.

Shi Zhong Ru (**Stalactitum**)[53] is sweet and warm. It mainly treats cough and counterflow qi ascent. It brightens the eyes, boosts the essence, quiets the five viscera, frees the hundreds of joints, disinhibits the nine orifices, and promotes lactation. It is produced in mountains and valleys.

Yin Nie (**Stalactitum**) is acrid and warm. It mainly treats frostbite, blood stasis, diarrhea and dysentery, cold and heat, mouse fistulas, and concretion and conglomeration bound qi. Its other name is *Jiang Shi* (Ginger Stone). It is produced in mountains and valleys.

Kong Gong Nie (**Stalactitum**) is acrid and warm. It mainly treats food damage, nontransformation of food, evil bound qi, malign sores, flat

---

[52] This medicinal is toxic and erosive. It is only used to treat tooth decay, nasal polyps, sores, and flat abscesses. Occasionally, it is applied to eye diseases.

[53] This medicinal is obtained from the root of a stalactite. In differentiating *Shi Zhong Ru* and the next two medicinals, Li Shi-zhen, the great Ming dynasty pharmacologist, explains that a stalactite is like a breast. The nipple is *Shi Zhong Ru*, the body is *Kong Gong Nie*, and the root is *Yin Nie*.

abscesses, and hemorrhoids and fistulas. It disinhibits the nine orifices and promotes lactation. It is produced in mountains and valleys.

Ci Huang (Auripigmentum) is acrid and balanced. It mainly treats malign sores, baldness, and scabs. It kills toxic insects and lice [causing] itching of the body, and [it treats] evil qi and all toxins. Protracted taking after it is sublimated may make the body light, prolong life, and prevent senility. It is produced in mountains and valleys.

Shi Liu Huang (Sulphur)[54] is sour and warm. It is toxic, treating mainly genital erosion in females, flat abscesses, hemorrhoids, and malign blood. It fortifies the sinews and bones and cures baldness. It is able to transform rare matters like gold, silver, copper, and iron. It is produced in mountains and valleys.

Yang Qi Shi (Actinolitum) is sour and nontoxic. It mainly treats flooding and leaking,[55] breaking the blood in the uterus, and concretion and conglomeration bound qi. [It also treats] cold and heat, abdominal pain, infertility, and impotence, and it supplements insufficiency. Its other name is *Bai Shi* (White Stone). It is produced in the mountains and valleys of Qi Shan.[56]

---

[54] In olden times, Sulphur was also used to treat cold vacuity of the lower origin, original qi bordering on expiry, enduring cold diarrhea, spleen and stomach vacuity, and some fatal diseases. However, because it is toxic, one must stop taking it once the disease has been hit.

[55] Flooding and leaking is due to damage of *chong* and *ren* vessels. Flooding refers to sudden, profuse vaginal bleeding, while leaking refers to continual, usually scanty dribbling of blood from the vagina. Wiseman's term for *beng lou* is flooding and spotting. However, the Chinese *lou* means to leak. In this case, spotting is not a denotative translation but rather a gloss on the meaning. Since this is a yin yang term, we feel it is best to translate the words and not gloss the meaning in modern terms.

[56] Qi Shan is in the suburbs of Jinan, the capital of present-day Shandong Province.

Ning Shui Shi **(Calcareous Spar)**[57] is acrid and cold. It mainly treats generalized fever, concretion and accumulation evil qi in the abdomen, burning heat within the skin, and vexatious fullness. It is taken with water. Protracted taking may make one free from hunger. Its other name is *Bai Shui Shi* (White Water Stone). It is produced in mountains and valleys.

Ci Shi **(Magnetitum)**[58] is acrid and cold. It mainly treats generalized impediment due to cold dampness, pain in the limb joints, inability to grip things, and continual soreness and aching. It eliminates great fever, vexatious fullness, and deafness. Its other name is *Xuan Shi* (Red Stone). It is produced in mountains and valleys.

Li Shi **(Gypsum Fibrosum)**[59] is acrid and cold. It mainly treats generalized fever, disinhibits the stomach, resolves vexation, boosts the essence, brightens the eyes, breaks accumulations and gatherings, and removes the three [kinds of] worms. Its other name is *Li Zhi Shi* (Instantly Ready Stone). It is produced in mountains and valleys.

Chang Shi **(Feldspar)** is acrid and cold. It mainly treats generalized fever and reversal cold of the limbs. It disinhibits urination, frees the flow of the blood vessels, brightens the eyes, eliminates screen causing blindness, removes the three [kinds of] worms, and kills *gu* toxins. Protracted taking may make one free of hunger. Its other name is *Fang Shi* (Rectangular Stone). It is produced in mountains and valleys.

---

[57] The pharmacological identification of this medicinal is still under some debate. Some authorities identify it as Glauberitum, Gypsum, or Calcitum.

[58] This medicinal is able to boost the kidney qi and supplement the essence and marrow. Therefore, it is used to treat kidney vacuity deafness and blurred vision.

[59] Although this medicinal's identity is not absolutely certain, it is probably either Gypsum or Calcitum.

11

Fu Qing (**Azuritum**)[60] is acrid. It mainly treats *gu* toxins, snake toxins, and all toxins of vegetables and meats as well as malign wounds.[61] Its other name is *Tui Qing* (Pushing Green-blue). It is produced in mountains and valleys.

Tie Luo (**Frusta Ferri**)[62] is acrid and balanced. It mainly treats wind heat, malign wounds, sores, flat abscesses, scabs, and [evil] qi within the skin. *Tie* (Ferrum) mainly fortifies the sinews and cultivates endurance to pain. *Tie Jing* (Frusta Ferri)[63] mainly brightens the eyes and is able to transform copper. [Ferrum] is produced in plains and swamps.

---

[60] This medicinal may also be Malachitum. Its identity is not certain.

[61] The word *chuang* has more than a single English meaning. Therefore, malign wound (*e chuang*) may also refer to malign sores.

[62] Chen Cang-qi, who lived in the 8th century CE, gave a detailed explanation about the indications of iron dust when he said:

It resolves various toxic substances having entered the abdomen, and, after being taken, it is able to settle the heart and brighten the eyes. Its indications include withdrawal and epilepsy, fever, acute jaundice, running about frenetically, and withdrawal and mania of the six kinds of domesticated animals. If a person is bitten by a snake, dog, tiger, wolf, or poisonous malign insects, one may take it and it will keep the toxins from penetrating.

[63] According to the text, there is a distinction between *Tie* (iron), *Tie Jing* (iron dust in the forge), and *Tie Luo* (iron dust fallen from the anvil while the iron is being struck). In some versions of this book, these three substances are treated in three separate passages. In other versions, these three are dealt with in a single passage as above.

Jades and Stones: Inferior Class

Shi Gao (Gypsum)[64] is acrid and slightly cold. It mainly treats wind stroke cold and heat, counterflow qi below the heart, fright, panting, dry mouth, parched tongue, inability to catch one's breath, and hardness and pain in the abdomen. It eliminates evil ghosts, promotes lactation, and [heals] incised wounds. It is produced in mountains and valleys.

Qing Lang Gan (Malachitum)[65] is acrid and balanced. It mainly treats itching of the body, burns, welling abscesses, sores, scabs, and dead muscles. Its other name is *Shi Zhu* (Stone Pearl). It is produced in plains and swamps.

Yu Shi (Arsenolitum)[66] is acrid. It is toxic, treating mainly cold and heat, mouse fistulas, erosion sores, dead muscles, wind impediment, hardness in the abdomen, and evil qi. It eliminates heat. Its other name is *Qing Fen Shi* (Green-blue Breakable Stone). Yet another name is *Li Zhi Shi* (Instantly

---

[64] In ancient times, Gypsum Fibrosum, which is presently called *Shi Gao*, was called *Li Shi*, while Gypsum, which was called *Shi Gao* in ancient times, is the present-day *Ying Shi Gao* (literally, Hard Gypsum). Fibrous Gypsum is particularly able to clear fire, including both stomach fire and lung fire, and to relax the spleen and boost the qi. Therefore, it is used to treat *yang ming* headache, cold and heat, tidal fever, intense thirst and massive drinking, summerheat, and toothache. Externally, it is often used to remove putrefied muscle (*i.e.*, flesh and skin), promote the growth of the muscles (*i.e.*, the flesh and skin), and stop pain.

[65] This medicinal may possibly be turquois.

[66] The identity of this medicinal is controversial. Some people suggest it is really Mispickel, while others reject this notion. In many other versions, there is "and greatly hot" after the word "acrid."

13

Ready Stone). It is also called *Gu Yang Shi* (Fasten Goat Stone). It is produced in mountains and valleys.

Dai Zhe (**Haematitum**) is bitter and cold. It mainly treats demonic influx, bandit wind,[67] and *gu* toxins. It kills spiritual matters and vicious ghosts as well as toxic and evil qi in the abdomen. It [checks] red ooze[68] and leaking. Its other name is *Xu Wan* (Hairy Pills). It is produced in mountains and valleys.

Lu Xian (**Alkali**)[69] is bitter, salty, and cold. It mainly treats great fever, wasting thirst, and manic vexation. It eliminates evils and [treats] vomiting and diarrhea and *gu* toxins. It softens [*i.e.*, makes elastic and flexible] the muscles and flesh.

Da Yan (**Sal**) causes people to vomit. *Rong Yan* (Halitum) brightens the eyes, [relieves] eye pain, boosts the qi, fortifies the muscles and bones, and eliminates *gu* toxins. These are produced in lakes and swamps.

---

[67] Wind can be either internal or external. Internal wind is generated within the body by, for instance, great heat, while external wind refers to the wind in nature. Bandit wind refers to external wind which causes disease. Another interpretation suggests that bandit wind refers to painful impediment.

[68] *Chi wo* (red ooze) usually means red dysentery. Since it is mentioned in juxtaposition with leaking and is clearly a female trouble, the translator suspects that here it refers to either vaginal or urethral bleeding.

[69] The author discusses Alkali, Salt and Halite in a single passage but gives different indications to each. Chen Cang-qi gave an account of the indications of Salt. He said:

It mainly treats red eyes, ulcered canthi, and wind ulceration of the eyelid rim. [For that purpose,] grind the Salt finely, mix it with water, and drop into the eye. [Salt] is able to enter the abdomen to eliminate heat, vexation, and phlegm fullness. [Besides, it treats] headache, brightens the eyes, and settles the heart. [For these purposes,] take it after grinding it in water. In addition, it mainly treats roundworms, snake and malign insect toxins, scabs, lichen, welling abscesses and swellings, and scrofulas.

Bai Wu (**Kaolin, Chalk**)[70] is bitter and warm. It mainly treats females' cold and heat, concretions and conglomerations, menstrual block [*i.e.*, amenorrhea], accumulations and gatherings, genital swelling and pain, leaking, and infertility. It is produced in mountains and valleys.

Qian Dan (**Minium**) is acrid and slightly cold. It mainly treats cough and counterflow, stomach reflux,[71] fright epilepsy, and madness. It eliminates heat and downbears the qi. When sublimated, it turns back into *Jiu Guang* (Nine Lights).[72] Protracted taking may enable one to communicate with the spirit light. It is produced in plains and swamps.

Fen Xi (**Galenitum Praeparatum**) is acrid and cold. It mainly treats hidden corpse[73] and toxic [insect] bites. It kills the three [kinds of] worms.

---

[70] Chalk is also used to treat vacuity heat stomach reflux, diarrhea, nosebleed, hemorrhoids, and, externally, sores on the lower leg, genital itching, and head sores.

[71] Stomach reflux refers to vomiting in the evening what was eaten in the morning or, in the morning, what was eaten the previous evening. When extreme, there is vomiting on eating. This is often complicated by a hard mass below the heart and alternating cold and heat.

[72] The meaning of the term Nine Lights is difficult to determine. Some people suspect that it is a medicine in pill form. However, the translator does not think this is plausible.

[73] Hidden corpse is a disease characterized by spells of pricking pain in the heart region and abdomen with swelling and distention as well as panting for breath. However, when the spell is gone, the patient returns to normal. This is believed to be caused by a hidden evil which has lain for a long time deep in the five viscera. According to Ri Hua-zi, who lived in the early years of the Song dynasty, so called hidden corpse might imply swollen welling abscesses, counterflow vomiting, concretions and conglomerations, and *gan*. *Gan* is a disease commonly seen in children whose main characteristic is indigestion and emaciation.

15

Xi Tong Jing Bi (Compound of Tin & Copper)[74] mainly treats females' blood block, concretions and conglomerations lying in the intestines, and infertility. [Galenite] is also named *Jie Xi* (Disintegratable Tin). It is produced in the mountains and valleys of Gui Yang.[75]

Shi Hui (Limestone) is acrid and warm. It mainly treats flat abscesses, scabs, heat qi, malign sores, *lai* disease,[76] dead muscles, and falling eyebrows. It kills hemorrhoidal worms[77] and eliminates black moles and polyps. Its other name is *Wu Hui* (Chalk Lime). It is produced in mountains and valleys.

Dong Hui (Pulvis Fumi Carbonisati)[78] is acrid and slightly warm. It mainly treats black moles and eliminates polyps and warts, flat abscesses, erosive [sores], and scabs. Its other name is *Li Hui* (Chenopodium Ash).

---

[74] This was a compound of lead and copper from which mirrors were made in olden times. In those times, tin was often confused with lead.

[75] *I.e.,* present-day Chenzhou, Hunan Province

[76] This refers to leprosy.

[77] The translator has failed to identify hemorrhoidal worms. This term may refer to pinworms. This sentence may also mean healing hemorrhoids and killing parasites.

[78] This is simply plant ash. However, the ash of *Hui Di Cai* (Herba Chenopodii Serotini) is regarded as the best of all. Therefore, at the end of this passage this medicinal is given the name of Chenopodium Ash.

Herbs: Superior Class

Qing Zhi **(Ganoderma Viridis)**[79] is sour and balanced. It mainly brightens the eyes, supplements the liver qi, quiets the essence and ethereal soul, and [cultivates] humanity and compassion. Protracted taking may make the body light, prevent senility, and prolong life so as to make one an immortal. Its other name is *Long Zhi* (Dragon Ganoderma). It grows in mountains and valleys.

Chi Zhi **(Ganoderma Rubra)** is bitter and balanced. It mainly treats binding in the chest, boosts the heart qi, supplements the center, sharpens the wits, and [causes people] not to forget [*i.e.*, improves the memory]. Protracted taking may make the body light, prevent senility, and prolong life so as to make one an immortal. Its other name is *Dan Zhi* (Cinnabar Ganoderma). It grows in mountains and valleys.

Huang Zhi **(Ganoderma Aurea)** is sweet and balanced. It mainly treats the five evils in the heart and abdomen,[80] boosts the spleen qi, quiets the

---

[79] In this book, Ganoderma is divided into six types depending on its color. Because Ganoderma is one of the best medicinals, it is called Immortal Weed. It is not only able to prevent and treat disease but is said to even cultivate virtues.

[80] There are several different interpretations of the five evils. They may either be pathogens of the five viscera; wind stroke, summerheat damage, food, drink, and taxation fatigue, cold damage, and dampness stroke; wind, cold, dampness, fog, and food damage; or vacuity, repletion, bandit, mild, and regular evils. In this context, probably this last group is what is meant. So-called bandit evils refer to a disease caused by a pathogen pertaining to the restraining phase. For example, if heart fire becomes diseased due to kidney water, this is a bandit evil. Regular evils refer to visceral disease caused only by the involved viscus itself. Mild evils refer to a disease caused by an evil pertaining to the restrained phase. If heart disease is transmitted from the lung metal, then this is a so-called mild evil.

spirit, and [cultivates] loyalty, honesty, gentleness, and a carefree mind. Protracted taking may make the body light, prevent senility, and prolong life so as to make one an immortal. Its other name is *Jin Zhi* (Gold Ganoderma). It grows in mountains and valleys.

Bai Zhi (Ganoderma Alba) is acrid and balanced. It mainly treats cough and counterflow qi ascent, boosts the lung qi, disinhibits the mouth and nose, fortifies the will [to cultivate] bravery and undauntedness, and quiets the corporeal soul. Protracted taking may make the body light, prevent senility, and prolong life so as to make one an immortal. Its other name is *Yu Zhi* (Jade Ganoderma). It grows in mountains and valleys.

Hei Zhi (Ganoderma Nigra) is salty and balanced. It mainly treats urinary dribbling block, disinhibits the water passageways, boosts the kidney qi, frees the nine orifices, and sharpens the hearing. Protracted taking may make the body light, prevent senility, and prolong life so as to make one an immortal. Its other name is *Xuan Zhi* (Dark Ganoderma). It grows in mountains and valleys.

Zi Zhi (Ganoderma Purpurea)[81] is sweet and warm. It mainly treats deafness, disinhibits the joints, protects the spirit, boosts the essence qi, fortifies the sinews and bones, and renders a good facial complexion. Protracted taking may make the body light, prevent senility, and prolong life so as to make one an immortal. Its other name is *Mu Zhi* (Wood Ganoderma). It grows in mountains and valleys.

---

[81] All the different kinds of Ganoderma except for Purple Ganoderma are explained according to five phase theory. Take White Ganoderma for example. White corresponds to metal which, in turn, corresponds to the lungs. Therefore, it supplements the lung qi, boosts the corporeal soul, and is able to disinhibit the qi track [*i.e.*, the respiratory track], the nose, and mouth. Purple Ganoderma is the only Ganoderma not discussed in this way. Based on this, the suspicion arises that Purple Ganoderma was added by some later editor(s).

Tian Men Dong (**Tuber Asparagi Cochinensis**)[82] is bitter and balanced. It mainly treats all sudden wind dampness and hemilateral impediment.[83] It strengthens the bone marrow, kills the three [kinds of] worms, and removes the hidden corpse. Protracted taking may make the body light, boost the qi, and prolong life. Its other name is *Dian Le* (Curb at the Top). It grows in mountains and valleys.

Zhu (**Rhizoma Atractylodis**)[84] is bitter and warm. It mainly treats damp impediment, dead muscles, tetany, and jaundice. It stops sweating, eliminates heat, and disperses food. It can be used as a conductor in decoctions. Protracted taking may make the body light, prolong life, and make one free from hunger.[85] Its other name is *Shan Ji* (Mountain Thistle). It grows in the mountains and valleys of Zheng Shan.[86]

---

[82] Asparagus is actually bitter in flavor and cold of qi. Nowadays it is used to treat panting, steaming heat, ejection of blood, and vacuity taxation. In addition, it is good for moistening dry intestines. However, it is seldom used for wind dampness (*i.e.*, rheumatism). In olden times, Daoists regarded Asparagus as an important medicinal when composing supplementing formulas. For this purpose, it was usually combined with *Di Huang* (Radix Rehmanniae) and *Ren Shen* (Radix Panacis Ginseng). They were called Trinity of Heaven (Asparagus), Earth (Rehmannia), and Humanity (Ginseng).

[83] Hemilateral impediment sometimes means hemiplegia.

[84] Here, two medicinals are meant, *Cang Zhu* (Rhizoma Atractylodis) and *Bai Zhu* (Rhizoma Atractylodis Macrocephalae). In olden times, the former was called *Chi Zhu* (literally, Red Atractylodes), while the latter was called *Bai Zhu* (White Atractylodes). This latter term is still in use today. *Bai Zhu* (Rhizoma Atractylodis Macrocephalae) is able to harmonize the center and dry dampness and, therefore, is used to treat retching and vomiting, diarrhea, non-transformation of food, and taxation fatigue. Depending on which other medicinals it is combined with, it can either promote or stop sweating, quiet the fetus, supplement the blood, and boost the qi. *Cang Zhu* (Rhizoma Atractylodis) has similar effects but is drastically drying in nature. It is better for stopping sweating. In addition, it is often used to disperse swelling and fullness, resolve depression, and cure wilting (*i.e.*, atony).

[85] Making one free from hunger here simply implies that this medicinal can be used as a food.

[86] This is a place in the present-day Shaanxi Province.

Wei Rui (**Rhizoma Polyganati Odorati**)[87] is sweet and balanced. It mainly treats wind stroke with fulminant heat and inability to stir, sprained sinews, binding of flesh, and all insufficiency. Protracted taking may remove black patches from the face. It renders the facial complexion good and shiny, makes the body light, and prevents senility. It grows in rivers and valleys [or river valleys].

Gan Di Huang (**dry Radix Rehmanniae**)[88] is sweet and cold. It mainly treats broken [bones], severed sinews from falls, and damaged center. It expels blood impediment,[89] replenishes the bone marrow, and promotes the growth of muscles and flesh. When used in decoctions, it eliminates cold and heat, accumulations and gatherings, and impediment. Using the uncooked is better. Protracted taking may make the body light and prevent senility. Its other name is *Di Sui* (Earth Marrow). It grows in [*i.e.*, near] rivers and swamps.

---

[87] In olden times, this medicinal was often confused with *Wei Ling Xian* or *Nu Wan* (Radix Clematidis Chinensis). As a result, descriptions of its indications were sometimes confusing. Nowadays, it is used mainly as a supplementing medicinal to treat vacuity taxation, glomus, generalized heaviness, and difficult speech. In addition, it treats impediment of the limbs, dampness influx lumbago, tearing, and black spots on the face.

[88] This passage apparently includes dry, cooked, and uncooked Radix Rehmanniae. In modern prescriptions, dry Radix Rehmanniae is used to supplement yin and cool the blood to treat yin vacuity with internal heat, taxation cough, wilting, impediment, and fright palpitation. In addition, it treats fracture and severed sinews, quiets the fetus, and kills parasites. Uncooked Radix Rehmanniae (*Sheng Di Huang*) is bitter in flavor and cold of qi. It drains fire from the heart, kidneys, and intestines. It is an indispensable medicinal for treating diseases involving the blood. Cooked Radix Rehmanniae (*Shu Di Huang*) is sweet and warm. It enriches kidney water and promotes the generation of blood and marrow. It is particularly good for taxation damage.

[89] Blood impediment is a species of impediment manifesting as insensitivity of the limbs and pain in the limb joints. It is due to wind cold invading and congesting the vessels as a result of vacuity and sweating in a draft during sleep. It is sometimes used as a synonym for wind impediment.

Chang Pu (**Rhizoma Acori Graminei**)[90] is acrid and warm. It mainly treats wind cold damp impediment and cough and counterflow qi ascent. It opens the heart portals, supplements the five viscera, frees the nine orifices, brightens the eyes and [sharpens] the hearing, and [helps] the articulation of the voice. Protracted taking may make the body light, improve memory, prevent confusion, and prolong life. Its other name is *Chang Yang* (Flourishing Yang). It grows in pools and swamps.

Yuan Zhi (**Radix Polygalae Tenuifoliae**)[91] is bitter and warm. It mainly treats cough with counterflow and damaged center, supplements insufficiency, eliminates evil qi, disinhibits the nine orifices, sharpens the wits, brightens the eyes and [sharpens] the hearing, improves memory, strengthens the will, and doubles [one's physical] strength. Protracted taking may make the body light and prevent senility. The leaves [*i.e.*, Folium Polygalae Tenuifoliae] are called *Xiao Cao* (Small Weed). Its other name is *Ji Wan* (Bramble). Yet another name is *Yao Rao* (Twining). It is also called *Xi Cao* (Thin Weed). It grows in rivers and valleys.

---

[90] Acorus is able to eliminate cold water, disperse phlegm rheum, and dissipate blood stasis. Therefore, it is prescribed to treat all kinds of wind disease, including obstinate impediment of the limbs and paralysis. It also opens the stomach, harmonizes the blood, secures the teeth, brightens the eyes, opens the heart orifice, and treats the five taxations and seven damages.

[91] Polygala is also able to transform phlegm and heal both welling and flat abscesses. Liao Xi-yong (1556-1627? CE) said:

Welling and flat abscesses are both the result of depressed seven affects and anger and indignation. Polygala is acrid and, therefore, able to dissipate depression. This is why it is capable of treating welling and flat abscesses.

Ze Xie **(Rhizoma Alismatis)**[92] is sweet and cold. It mainly treats wind, cold, damp impediment and difficult lactation. It disperses water, nourishes the five viscera, boosts the qi and [physical] force, and makes one fat and strong. Protracted taking may sharpen the ears and eyes, make one free from hunger, prolong life, make the body light, render the face brilliant, and enable one to walk over water. Its other name is *Shui Xie* (Water Drain). Yet another name is *Mang Yu* (Awned Yam). It is also called *Hu Xie* (Swan Drain). It grows in pools and swamps.

Shu Yu **(Radix Dioscoreae Oppositae)** is sweet and a little warm. It mainly treats damaged center, supplements vacuity with languor, eliminates cold and heat and evil qi, supplements the center, boosts the qi and energy, and promotes the growth of the muscles and flesh. Protracted taking may sharpen the ears and eyes, make the body light, make one free from hunger, and prolong life. Its other name is *Shan Yu* (Mountain Yam). It grows in mountains and valleys.

---

[92]   Alisma is an important medicinal for percolating dampness and disinhibiting water. It is a bit salty; so it is capable of penetrating the kidneys. Zhang Zhi-cong (1610-1674? CE) gave a detailed annotation to this passage saying:

> The reason why it mainly treats wind, cold, damp impediment is its ability to bring up the water fluids from the lower part to irrigate the interstices of the flesh and skin through center earth. Breast milk is the fluid from the middle burner. When water fluids enrich center earth, difficult lactation is cured. The five viscera receive the essence from water and grain. Alisma can enrich center earth, so it is able to nourish the five viscera. The kidneys are organs which produce force. When water essence is upborne to supply nourishment, the qi force [i.e., physical strength] is boosted. When the interstices of the flesh are irrigated via the center, the person gains weight and becomes strong. Because water qi is able to ascend and then descend, water [swelling] is dispersed.

Ju Hua (**Flos Chrysanthemi Morifolii**)[93] is bitter and balanced. It mainly treats head wind, head dizziness, and head swelling and pain with the eyes [painful] as if they were fit to burst from their sockets, tearing, dead skin and muscles, aversion to wind, and damp impediment. Protracted taking may disinhibit the blood and qi, make the body light, slow aging, and prolong life. Its other name is *Jie Hua* (Seasonal Flower). It grows in rivers and swamps.

Gan Cao (**Radix Glycyrrhizae**)[94] is sweet and balanced. It mainly treats the five viscera and six bowels, cold and heat, and evil qi. It fortifies the sinews and bones, promotes the growth of the muscles and flesh, doubles [one's physical] strength, [heals] incised wounds and swellings, and resolves toxins. Protracted taking may make the body light and prolong life. It grows in rivers and valleys.

---

[93] Chrysanthemum is able to supplement water and boost metal. Once metal is brought to order, wood is automatically levelled. Once wood is levelled, wind will subside and fire will be eliminated. For that reason, Chrysanthemum is prescribed to treat damp impediment, wandering wind, and wind headache and wind dizziness. Wind headache and dizziness accompany one another. This syndrome attacks unpredictably and irregularly just as wind does. During an attack, there is dizziness often complicated by headache, blurred vision, counterflow vomiting, and, in extreme cases, reversal cold of the limbs. In addition, Chrysanthemum supplements yin blood. Once the blood is settled and the liver is levelled, eye diseases are cured.

[94] Wang Ang (1615-17?? CE) said:

Used uncooked, Licorice supplements spleen and stomach insufficiency and drains heart fire. After being mix-fried, it supplements the triple burner original qi and dissipates exterior cold. Put in a harmonizing formula, it supplements and boosts. Put in a sweating formula, it resolves the muscles. Put in a cooling formula, it drains evil heat. Put in a precipitating formula, it moderates the righteous qi. Put in a moistening formula, it nourishes the yin blood. It is able to coordinate with various medicinals preventing them from clashing with each other. It promotes the growth of the muscles, relieves pain, and resolves the toxins of various medicinals.

Ren Shen (**Radix Panacis Ginseng**)[95] is sweet and a little cold. It mainly supplements the five viscera. It quiets the essence spirit, settles the ethereal and corporeal souls, checks fright palpitations, eliminates evil qi, brightens the eyes, opens the heart, and sharpens the wits. Protracted taking may make the body light and prolong life. Its other name is *Ren Xian* (Human

[95] Based on this work, Li Gao, a.k.a Li Dong-yuan (1180-1251 CE), gave a general analysis of the actions of Ginseng. He said, "Ginseng drains fire, quiets the spirit, stabilizes the corporeal soul, fortifies the spleen, brightens the eyes, eliminates vexatious thirst, breaks hardness and gathering, and treats vacuity taxation internal damage and all blood illnesses." From this account, it is obvious that Ginseng is a multi-purpose medicinal. As far as its fire-draining function is concerned, it can be applied in many ways. Together with Cimicifuga, it drains lung fire. With the help of Poria, it drains kidney fire. When combined with Ophiopogon and Schisandra, it generates the vessels (*i.e.*, the pulse). And it is able to abate intense fever when prescribed together with Licorice and Astragalus.

In regard to its indications and contraindications, Jiang Ju-zhi, who lived in the Qing dynasty, said in his *Ben Cao Zhai Yao Gang Mu (Outlined Extractions from the Materia Medica)*:

White, yellow, or green-blue dusty facial complexion with a haggard [look] reveals insufficiency of the spleen, lungs, or kidneys. [In that case, Ginseng] is indicated. Red or black facial complexion shows vigorous qi and strong spirit. [In that case,] Ginseng is prohibited [*i.e.*, contraindicated]. If the pulse is floating as well as scallion-stalk and soggy; is vacuous and large; is slow, moderate, and forceless; is deep and slow; or is choppy; weak; thin; bound; or regularly interrupted and forceless, this shows vacuity and insufficiency. [Then Ginseng] is indicated. If the pulse is bowstring and long; tight; replete; slippery; or rapid and forceful, this is a result of fire depression and internal repletion. [In that case,] Ginseng is prohibited. In case of panting and coughing, Ginseng should not be used. In case of kidney vacuity and rough breathing with shortness of breath, it should be prescribed without delay. If cough is produced by cold embracing heat evils which are congested in the lungs, it is prohibited. If spontaneous sweating and aversion to cold accompany cough with disharmony of the central qi, it should be used without delay. In case of enduring disease where heat is depressed in the lungs, it is prohibited. When there is lung vacuity with effulgent fire causing shortness of breath and spontaneous sweating, it must be used. In various kinds of pain, it should not be used imprudently. In case of internal vacuity vomiting and diarrhea or in case of enduring disease where the stomach is vacuous and weak and thus giving rise to pain which is relievable by pressure, it must be used.

Incarnation). Yet another name is *Gui Gai* (Ghost Shield). It grows in mountains and valleys.

Shi Hu (Herba Dendrobii)[96] is sweet and balanced. It mainly treats damaged center. It eliminates impediment, downbears the qi, supplements the five viscera and vacuity taxation with languor and emaciation, and fortifies yin. Protracted taking may thicken [*i.e.*, fortify] the stomach and intestines, make the body light, and prolong life. Its other name is *Lin Lan* (Wood Orchid). It grows in mountains and valleys.

Shi Long Rui (Semen Ranunculi Sclerati) is bitter and balanced. It mainly treats wind cold damp impediment and evil qi in the heart and abdomen. It disinhibits the joints and stops vexatious fullness. Protracted taking may make the body light, brighten the eyes, and prevent senility. Its other name is *Lu Neng Guo* (Lu's Able Fruit). Yet another name is *Di Ren* (Earth Mulberry). It grows in rivers and swamps.

---

[96] Dendrobium is particularly able to supplement the spleen and stomach to eliminate vacuity heat and generate fluids. In order to gain a better understanding of some of the technical terms in this passage, the following quote from Zhang Zhi-cong may be useful:

When dealing with the indications of the superior class, the *Ben Jing* usually merely mentions elimination of impediment instead of wind, cold, and dampness. Mere mention of impediment implies that [this category of] impediment is an exterior [disorder] related to the five viscera. The skin is related to the lungs. The vessels are related to the heart. The flesh is related to the spleen. The sinews are related to the liver. The bones are related to the kidneys. To eliminate impediment, one should treat vacuity and taxation, languor and emaciation due to the five viscera. Thus one may achieve the miraculous effect of supplementing and boosting while [Dendrobium] is made to attack the evils in the center. Downbearing the qi through treating the damaged center is carrying out [downbearing] along with supplementation and boosting. Here lies a divine principle of attacking evils.

Niu Xi (**Radix Achyrathis Bidentatae**)[97] is bitter and balanced. It mainly treats cold damp wilting and impediment, hypertonicity of the limbs, and pain in the knees with inability to bend or stretch. It expels the blood and qi,[98] [treats] heat damage and burns, and induces abortion. Protracted taking may make the body light and slow aging. Its other name is *Bai Bei* (Hundredfold). It grows in rivers and valleys.

Xi Xin (**Herba Asari Cum Radice**)[99] is acrid and a little warm. It mainly treats cough and counterflow, headache and shaking brain, hypertonicity of the hundreds of joints, wind damp impediment and pain, and dead muscles. It brightens the eyes and disinhibits the nine orifices. Protracted

---

[97] When processed with wine, Achyranthes boosts the liver and kidneys and fortifies the sinews and bones. Therefore, it is able to treat foot wilting, hypertonicity of the sinews, pain in the lumbus, knees, and bones, impotence, enuresis, enduring malaria, dysentery, damaged center and diminished qi, severe pain in the heart and abdomen, strangury and hematuria, amenorrhea, and difficult delivery. If it is used unprocessed, it dissipates the blood, resolves binding, and breaks concretions and conglomerations. Achyranthes is also able to lead fire downward and conduct various medicinals downward towards the feet. However, because of this action, it should not be used in cases of spleen qi vacuity sunken below. Otherwise, it may give rise to troubles like seminal emission.

[98] Expelling the blood and qi implies breaking binding and dispersing concretions and conglomerations.

[99] Asarum is particularly strong for removing wind cold. Zou Shu (1790-1844 CE) said:

Whenever wind qi and cold qi cling to the essence, blood, and fluids so as to give rise to troubles related to urination, snivel, and sputum, [Asarum] can drain and drive them out...As discussed in the *Ben Jing*, it is able to treat cough and counterflow [as a result of wind cold clinging to rheum in the chest], headache and shaking brain [as a result of wind cold clinging to the brain marrow], hypertonicity of the hundreds of joints [as a result of wind cold clinging to the humors in the joints], and wind damp impediment pain and dead muscles [as a result of wind cold clinging to the fluids in the muscles and flesh]...

Asarum boosts the liver and gallbladder. Therefore, it is able to treat fright epilepsy, tearing on exposure to wind, and binding.

taking may make the body light and prolong life. Its other name is *Xiao Xin* (Small Acrid). It grows in mountains and valleys.

Du Huo **(Radix Angelicae Pubescentis)** is bitter and balanced. It is nontoxic, treating mainly assaulting wind cold and incised wounds. It relieves pain, running piglet, epilepsy, and tetany, and, in females, mounting conglomeration. Protracted taking may make the body light and slow aging. Its other name is *Qiang Huo* (Qiang Activator).[100] Yet another name is *Qiang Qing* (Qiang Green-blue). It is also called *Hu Qiang Shi Zhe* (Protecting the Qiang Envoy). It grows in rivers and valleys.

Sheng Ma **(Rhizoma Cimicifugae)**[101] is sweet and balanced. It mainly resolves the hundreds of toxins, kills the hundreds of essence, old matters, and ravaging ghosts,[102] and keeps off scourge epidemics, miasmic evils, and *gu* toxins. Protracted taking may prevent premature death, make the body light, and lengthen life. Its other name is *Zhou Sheng Ma* (Zhou's Cimicifuga). It grows in mountains and valleys.

---

[100] The Qiang were a tribe of nomads living in northwest China in olden times.

[101] The main actions of Cimicifuga include upbearing the clear and downbearing the turbid, resolving toxins and repulsing epidemic qi. To upbear the clear and downbear the turbid, it is used in combination with Chinese Scallion. To dissipate wind evils from the *yang ming* channel, it is used together with Gypsum. When it is used together with Bupleurum, Ginseng, and Atragalus, it leads them upward to relieve toothache. With its help, Pueraria is able to promote sweat in *yang ming* patterns. In addition, it is often used to treat spleen vacuity. Zhang Yuan-su, who lived in the Jin dynasty (1115-1234 CE) said:

> Without it as an usher, spleen-supplementing medicinals cannot bring any effect. Spleen impediment cannot be removed unless it is used.

[102] So-called essence which here means spirit, old materials, and ravaging ghosts all refer to various sorts of sudden diseases with generalized symptoms usually complicated by mental disorders. It was believed in ancient China that anything having grown to an extraordinarily old age will produce a special spirit. An age-old tree, for example, might have a spirit dwelling in it. This would be called tree spirit. If this spirit was ill-tempered by nature or if someone did something insulting to it, the person might suffer.

27

Chai Hu (**Radix Bupleuri**)[103] is bitter and balanced. It mainly treats bound qi in the heart, abdomen, intestines, and stomach, drink and food accumulation and gathering, cold and heat, and evil qi. It weeds out the stale to bring forth the new. Protracted taking may make the body light, brighten the eyes, and boost the essence. Its other name is *Di Xun* (Earth Fuming). It grows in rivers and valleys.

Fang Kui (**Radix Peucedani Japonici**) is acrid and cold. It mainly treats mounting conglomeration, diarrhea, heat bound in the bladder causing urinary stoppage, cough and counterflow, warm malaria, epilepsy, fright evil, and manic running about. Protracted taking may fortify the bone marrow, boost the qi, and make the body light. Its other name is *Li Gai* (Pear Cover). It grows in rivers and valleys.

Chu Shi (**Fructus Ailanthi Altissimi**) is bitter and balanced. It mainly treats impotence, boosts the qi, replenishes the skin and muscles, brightens the eyes, and [makes one] wise and intelligent so as to forsee [the future]. Protracted taking may make one free from hunger, prevent senility, and make the body light. It grows in mountains and valleys.

---

[103] In regard to the actions of Bupleurum, the words of Ye Gui (1667-1746 CE) are instructive:

> The viscera and bowels together have 12 channels. All the 11 organs rely on the gallbladder for decision-making. Bupleurum is able to lift and set free the gallbladder qi. So long as the gallbladder qi reaches in an orderly [manner], the [other] 11 organs are in good order and are able to effuse and transform. As a result, any bound qi, be it in the heart or abdomen, the stomach or intestines, will be dispersed.

Of all the formulas containing Bupleurum, *Da Xiao Chai Hu Tang* (Major/Minor Bupleurum Decoctions) are the most famous and most widely used. In these formulas, Bupleurum is used to treat both the blood and qi. It may lead the clear qi of the *yang ming* up. In the treatment of cold damage or miscellaneous diseases, these formulas may resolve exterior cold, muscle heat, and alternating cold and heat, and, in females, cure blood entering the blood chamber and irregular menstruation. Besides, they are able to disperse blood binding and qi gathering.

An Lu Zi **(Herba Artemisiae Keiskeanae)**[104] is bitter and a little warm. It is nontoxic, treating mainly blood stasis in the five viscera, water qi in the abdomen, abdominal distention, persisting heat, wind cold damp impediment, and various kinds of pain in the body. Protracted taking may make the body light, prolong life, and prevent senility. It grows in rivers and valleys.

Yi Yi Ren **(Semen Coicis Lachryma-jobi)**[105] is sweet and slightly cold. It mainly treats hypertonicity of the sinews with inability to contract or stretch and wind damp impediment.[106] It downbears. Protracted taking may make the body light and boost the qi. Its root [*i.e.*, Radix Coicis Lachryma-jobi] is able to precipitate the three [kinds of] worms. Its other name is *Jie Li* (Woodworm Eliminator). It grows in plains and swamps.

Che Qian Zi **(Herba Plantaginis)** is sweet and cold. It is nontoxic, mainly treating qi dribbling urinary block. It relieves pain, disinhibits the water passageways and [hence] urination, and eliminates damp impediment. Protracted taking may make the body light and slow aging. Its other name is *Dang Dao* (Obstacle on the Road). It grows in plains and swamps.

---

[104] Artemisia is good at moving water and dissipating stasis, incorporating supplementation with dissipation, and is, therefore, able to treat impotence, pain in the lumbus, knee, and other joints, postpartum blood and qi pain, and fracture and sprain.

[105] Coix is a medicinal for center earth, but it also enters the lungs and liver. In short, it fortifies the spleen and boosts the stomach. When earth is made strong, metal will also become strong. Therefore, Coix is able to treat lung wilting and lung abscess. So long as earth is strong, water will not be aggressive. For that reason, Coix can treat water swelling and diarrhea. Diseases involving the sinews and bones are rooted in the *yang ming*. It follows that when there is sinew hypertonicity, impediment, and wilting, Coix may also be used. However, it should not be used for cold impediment because it is cold of qi. In addition, Coix treats wasting thirst, indigestion, heart and abdominal fullness, chest and rib-side pain, throat abscess, and toothache.

[106] It should be noted that cold impediment is excluded from Coix's indications because of its cold nature. However, in case of enduring cold impediment which has transformed into fire, Coix once again becomes an appropriate medicinal.

Xi Ming Zi (**Semen Thlaspi Arvensis**)[107] is acrid and slightly warm. It is nontoxic, mainly brightening the eyes, [treating] eye pain and tearing, eliminating impediment, supplementing the five viscera, and boosting the essence light. Protracted taking may make the body light and prevent senility. Its other name is *Bi Xin* (Grate Firewood). Yet another name is *Da Ji* (Great Tribulus). It is also called *Ma Xin* (Horse Acrid). It grows in mountains and swamps.

Chong Wei Zi (**Semen Leonuri Heterophylli**)[108] is acrid and slightly warm. It mainly brightens the eyes, boosts the essence, and eliminates water qi. Protracted taking may make the body light. The stalk [*i.e.*, Herba Leonuri Heterrophylli] mainly treats addictive itching papules.[109] It can [be used] to make bathwater [for newborns]. Its other name is *Yi Mu* (Mother Booster). Yet another name is *Yi Ming* (Brightness Booster). It is also called *Da Zha* (Great Armor Plate). It grows in pools and swamps.

---

[107] The identity of this medicinal is difficult to determine because many herbs have the same name. Therefore, its effects depicted here are questionable. In any case, this medicinal is seldom if ever used in modern times.

[108] The current name of this medicinal is *Yi Mu Cao* (Mother Boosting Herb). Leonurus quickens the blood, supplements yin, and boosts the qi. It is an important medicinal for treating women's diseases. Because it is able to supplement yin, it brightens the eyes and boosts the essence. Because it is able to quicken the blood, it regulates menstruation and treats postpartum troubles involving the blood. In addition, it treats mammary abscesses, sores, and nodes.

[109] This refers to nettle rash and other allergic skin rashes. Wiseman translates *yin zhen* as dormant papules. This Chinese term implies two characteristics of the papules. One is severe itching so that the patient is addicted to scratching them constantly. The other is its recurrence. While Wiseman's term dormant papules is derived from the fact that these types of rashes recur after periods of latency or dormancy, I prefer to stress the concept of addictive itching.

Mu Xiang (**Radix Auklandiae Lappae**)[110] is acrid and warm. It mainly treats evil qi, wards off toxic epidemics and warmth ghosts, and strengthens the will. It mainly treats rolling sweats.[111] Protracted taking may prevent oppressive ghost dreams in sleep either during the day or night. It grows in mountains and valleys.

Long Dan (**Radix Gentianae Scabrae**)[112] is bitter and astringent. It mainly treats cold and heat in the bones, fright epilepsy, and evil qi. It mends expiry and damage, settles the five viscera, and kills *gu* toxins. Protracted taking may sharpen the wits, improve the memory, make the body light,

---

[110] Auklandia is fragrant and, as such, it is a wonderful medicinal for nearly all kinds of qi troubles. Ni Zhu-mo of the Ming dynasty said in his *Ben Cao Hui Yan* (*Collection of the Commentaries on the Materia Medica*):

Auklandia harmonizes the stomach qi, frees the heart qi, downbears the lung qi, dredges the liver qi, quickens the spleen qi, warms the kidney qi, disperses accumulated qi, warms cold qi, normalizes counterflow qi, reaches exterior qi, and frees interior qi. In sum, it governs the various qi throughout the body, above and below, internally and externally. However, it is fragrant in flavor, dry in qi, and drastic in nature. [Therefore,] in case of lung vacuity with heat, desiccated blood with an agitated pulse, yin vacuity with upflaming fire, heart and stomach pain due to fire, vacuity and collapse of the original qi, and the various diseases with hidden heat, one should be careful not to use it.

Clinically, Auklandia is often used to treat the various kinds of heart pain, concretions and conglomerations, swelling and distention, choleraic disease, retching and vomiting, diarrhea, cold qi strings and aggregations, and dysentery.

[111] This refers to massive sweating due to being caught in the rain or affection by dew while staying out early in the morning or at night. There is, however, another interpretation according to which it means strangury or dribbling urination.

[112] Gentiana is bitter in flavor and cold of qi. The word astringent may be a typographical error. It is an important medicinal to drain fire from the liver and gallbladder. As such, it is able to brighten the eyes and cure jaundice caused by damp heat. Clinically, it is often used to treat fever, bone heat, abscesses and swellings, sores, scabs, roundworms, and, in children, fright epilepsy. It is also used for visiting hostility. This means a disease of sudden onset started by no identifiable cause and which is characterized by loss of consciousness, intense fever, and/or delirous speech.

31

and slow aging. Its other name is *Ling You* (Mound Ambling). It grows in mountains and valleys.

Tu Si Zi (**Semen Cuscutae Chinensis**)[113] is acrid and balanced. It mainly mends expiry and damage, supplements insufficiency, boosts the qi and [physical] strength, and makes one fat and strong. Protracted taking may brighten the eyes, make the body light, and prolong life. Its other name is *Tu Lu* (Rabbit Reed). It grows in mountains and valleys.

Ba Ji Tian (**Radix Morindae Officinalis**)[114] is acrid and slightly warm. It mainly treats great wind evil qi[115] and impotence, fortifies the sinews and bones, quiets the five viscera, supplements the center, improves the will, and boosts the qi. It grows in mountains and valleys.

Bai Mo (**Herba Solani Lyrati**)[116] is sweet and cold. It mainly treats cold and heat, the eight categories of jaundice,[117] and wasting thirst. It supplements the center and boosts the qi. Protracted taking may make the body light and prolong life. Its other name is *Gu Cai* (Grain Vegetable).

---

[113] Cuscuta is also used to treat vacuity cold and cold pain in the lumbus and knees, replenish the essence, and boost the marrow.

[114] Morinda is able to warm the liver and treat taxation damage, seminal emission, intercourse with ghosts in dreams, head wind, swollen feet, and impotence.

[115] Wind is the fiercest and most dangerous pathogen of all, and Morinda is able to conquer the worst wind.

[116] There is no consensus concerning the identity of this medicinal. Another possibility is that it is Herba Vincetoxici Atrati.

[117] Throughout the history of Chinese medicine, jaundice has been classified in different, confusing ways. Generally, it is divided into five types. The nine categories may be yellow, black, food, wine, sexual, acute, and fetal jaundice as well as yellow sweating.

Bai Hao (**Folium Artemisiae Argyi**)[118] is sweet and balanced. It mainly treats evil qi in the five viscera and wind cold damp impediment. It supplements the center, boosts the qi, promotes the growth of hair, is able to turn the hair black, and cures heart suspension which is [a syndrome including] reduced eating and constant hungering. Protracted taking may make the body light, sharpen the eyes and ears, and prevent senility. It grows in rivers and swamps.

Di Fu Zi (**Fructus Kochiae Scopariae**)[119] is bitter and cold. It mainly treats bladder heat, disinhibits urination, supplements the center, and boosts the essence qi. Protracted taking may sharpen the ears and eyes, make the body light, and slow aging. Its other name is *Di Kui* (Earth Big Flower). It grows in plains and swamps.

Shi Long Chu (**Herba Junci Baltici**) is bitter and slightly cold. It mainly treats evil qi in the heart and abdomen, inhibited urination, dribbling block, wind dampness, demonic influx, and [worm] malign toxins. Protracted taking may supplement vacuity with languor, make the body light, sharpen the ears and eyes, and prolong life. Its other name is *Long Xu* (Dragon's Beard). Yet another name is *Cao Xu Duan* (Herbaceous Dipsacus). It grows in mountains and valleys.

Luo Shi (**Folium Trachelospermi Jasminoidis**) is bitter and warm. It mainly treats wind heat, dead muscles, welling abscesses, wounds, dry mouth, parched tongue, refractory welling abscesses and swellings, swollen throat and tongue, and inability to take in [even] water. Protracted taking may make the body light, brighten the eyes, render the facial

---

[118] Artemisia Argyum is good for various women's diseases. It rectifies the qi and blood, removes cold dampness, regulates the menses, quiets the fetus, stops various kinds of bleeding, relieves abdominal pain and dysentery, and kills worms.

[119] This short passage summarizes all the actions of Kochia. In detail, it treats frequent urination, pain in urination, and dribbling urinary block as a result of frenetically stirring heat in the bladder. Because Kochia supplements the center and boosts the essence, it is able to cure impotence, troubles of the testicles, and lumbar pain. Externally, it can be used in the form of a washing solution. In that case, it treats various sorts of skin disease, including sores.

complexion good and shiny, prevent senility, and prolong life. Its other name is *Shi Ling* (Rock Bony Fish). It grows in rivers and valleys.

Huang Lian (Rhizoma Coptidis Chinensis)[120] is bitter. It is nontoxic, treating mainly heat qi, eye pain, injured canthi, and tearing. It brightens the eyes and [also treats] intestinal afflux, abdominal pain, dysentery, and, in females, genital swelling and pain. Protracted taking may improve the memory. Its other name is *Wang Lian* (King Lily). It grows in rivers and valleys.

Wang Bu Liu Xing (Semen Vacarriae Segetalis)[121] is bitter and balanced. It mainly treats incised wounds, stops bleeding, relieves pain, removes thorns, and eliminates wind impediment and internal cold. Protracted taking may make the body light, slow aging, and increase longevity. It grows in mountains and valleys.

---

[120] Coptis is very widely used in clinical practice. It enters the stomach, is able to dry dampness, and it eliminates heat. Therefore, it is used to drain heart fire, settle liver wind, and cool the blood. Because it is able to drain heart fire, it eliminates glomus and fullness in the chest and heart vexation due to heart fire. Because heart fire is also the cause of night sweats and some categories of sores, these also fall within the indications of Coptis. Chen Nian-zu (1753-1823 CE) said:

> When *The Classic* says it mainly treats heat qi, [it means that] it eliminates all heat in the qi division. Intestinal afflux, abdominal pain, and dysentery are all diseases [possibly] ascribed to damp heat in the center. Genital pain and swelling is an illness caused by damp heat below. Coptis eliminates damp heat. So these are all its indications.

[121] This medicinal is able to move the blood and treat wind toxins. Therefore, it is an important medicinal for the purpose of freeing the flow of the menses, promoting lactation, and hastening delivery.

Lan Shi (Semen Indigonis)[122] is bitter and cold. It mainly resolves various toxins and kills worms and infant ghost,[123] demonic influx, and insect bite toxins. Protracted taking may prevent the head hair from turning white and make the body light. It grows in plains and swamps.

Jing Tian (Herba Sedi Erythrosticti) is bitter, sour, and balanced. It mainly treats great fever, burns, generalized fever and vexation, and evil and malign qi. Its flower [*i.e.*, Flos Sedi Erythrosticti] mainly treats leaking and red and white [vaginal discharge] in females. It makes the body light and brightens the eyes. Its other name is *Jie Huo* (Fire Ban). Yet another name is *Shen Huo* (Fire Caution). It grows in rivers and valleys.

Tian Ming Jing (Herba Carpesii Abrotanoidis)[124] is sweet and cold. It mainly treats blood stasis and blood conglomeration bordering on death as well as blood precipitation. It stops bleeding, disinhibits urination, removes small worms, eliminates impediment, relieves bound heat in the chest, and quenches vexatious thirst. Protracted taking may make the body light and slow aging. Its other name is *Mai Ju Jiang* (Wheat Ginger). Yet another name is *Xia Mo Lan* (Frog Orchid). It is also called *Shi Shou* (Pig Head). It grows in rivers and swamps.

---

[122] This passage is very terse, yet pregnant with meaning. The short phrase, "resolving various toxins", for example, implies that, besides insect bites, etc. given in the text, this medicinal may treat clove toxins, wind papules, heat mania, swelling toxins, wandering wind heat toxins, heat *gan*, etc. Heat *gan* is a syndrome of vexatious heat in the five hearts, ulceration and reddening below the nose, sores on the head with dampness and itching, thirst and desire for water, yellow urine, and alternating cold and heat.

[123] This implies such fulminant diseases in children as high fever, fright wind, heat *gan* which manifests as low fever, dyspepsia, emaciation, enlarged abdomen, and diarrhea, and sudden disease with unidentified causes.

[124] Clinically, this medicinal is used to treat bleeding, phlegm malaria, toothache, acute and enduring fright wind, throat impediment, nipple moth (*i.e.*, tonsillitis), blood and sand strangury, and insect bite. In addition, it is a remedy for clenched jaw and faintness.

35

Pu Huang (**Pollen Typhae**)[125] is sweet and balanced. It mainly treats cold and heat related to the heart, abdomen, and urinary bladder. It disinhibits urination, stops bleeding, and disperses blood stasis. Protracted taking may make the body light, boost the qi and [physical] force, and prolong life so as to make one an immortal. It grows in pools and swamps.

Xiang Pu (**Herba Typhae Japonicae**) is sweet and balanced. It mainly treats evil qi in the five viscera and below the heart as well as putrefying mouth with foul smell. It fortifies the teeth, brightens the eyes, and sharpens the hearing. Protracted taking may make the body light and slow aging. Its other name is *Ju* (Osprey). It grows in pools and swamps.

Lan Cao (**Radix Eupatorii Chinensis**)[126] is acrid and balanced. It mainly disinhibits the water passageways, kills *gu* toxins, and keeps off ill matters.[127] Protracted taking may boost the qi, make the body light, slow aging, and enable one to communicate with the spirit light. Its other name is *Shui Xiang* (Water Fragrance). It grows in pools and swamps.

Jue Ming Zi (**Semen Cassiae Torae**) is salty and balanced. It mainly treats clear-eye blindness, spreading screen and red and white membrane in the eye, sore, red eyes, and tearing. Protracted taking may boost the essence light and make the body light. It grows in rivers and swamps.

---

[125] Pollen Typhae is a medicinal for the blood division of the hand and foot *jue yin*. Used uncooked, it is slippery in nature and, therefore, able to move the blood, disperse stasis, disinhibit urination, and eliminate cold and heat from the heart, abdomen, and bladder as well as postpartum vacuity vexation. Besides, it is often used to treat falls and knocks, sores, nodes, swelling, scrotal damp itch, distended tongue, tongue sores, and prolapse of the rectum. It can also be used charred. Then it becomes sluggish and, hence, is a wonderful medicinal to stop bleeding. This includes ejection of blood, hemafecia, hemorrhoidal bleeding, and bleeding wounds.

[126] The identity of this medicinal is controversial. Eupatorium Japonicum, Cymlidum Virens, Cymlidum Pumilum, etc. are all among the possibilities.

[127] It was believed that hanging this herb around one's dwelling on certain festivals might keep away unhappy events or mishaps.

Yun Shi (**Semen Caesalpiniae Sepiariae**) is acrid and a little warm. It mainly treats diarrhea and dysentery and intestinal afflux, kills worms and *gu* toxins, removes evil malign bound qi, relieves pain, and eliminates cold and heat. Its flower [*i.e.*, Flos Caesalpiniae Sepiariae] mainly treats seeing ghosts and spiritual matters. Taking much of it may make one run frenetically. Protracted taking may make the body light and enable one to communicate with the spirit light. It grows in rivers and valleys.

Huang Qi (**Radix Astragali Membranacei**)[128] is sweet and slightly warm. It mainly treats welling and flat abscesses and enduring festering sores [by] expelling pus and relieving pain, great wind *lai* disease, the five [kinds of] hemorrhoids,[129] and mouse fistulas. It supplements vacuity and [is good for] hundreds of diseases in children. Its other name is *Dai Sang* (Mulberry Cap). It grows in mountains and valleys.

She Chuang Zi (**Fructus Cnidii Monnieri**) is bitter and balanced. It mainly treats genital swelling and pain in females, and impotence and [genital] damp itch in males. It eliminates impediment qi, disinhibits the joints, and [treats] madness, epilepsy, and malign sores. Protracted taking may make the body light. Its other name is *She Su* (Snake Millet). Yet another name is *She Mi* (Snake Rice). It grows in rivers and valleys.

---

[128] Concerning the actions of Astragalus, Wang Hao-gu, a.k.a. Wang Hai-cang, an outstanding pupil of Li Gao and prolific medical writer, gave an instructive analysis when he said:

> Astragalus replenishes the defensive and, therefore, is a medicinal for the exterior. It boosts the spleen and stomach and, therefore, is a medicinal for the center. Since it is able to treat cold damage with the cubit pulse not arriving, it supplements the kidney origin and, hence, is a medicinal for the internal.

[129] The five kinds of hemorrhoids include female, male, vessel, intestinal, and blood. Female hemorrhoids are characterized by swelling and pustulation around the anus. Male hemorrhoids refers to a mouse fistula growing outside the anus which constantly gives off pus. Vessel hemorrhoids refer to splitting of the anus. While intestinal hemorrhoids are distinguished by swollen tubercles around the anus complicated by cold and heat and bleeding. Blood hemorrhoids are hemorrhoids with bleeding as the main sign.

Lou Lu (**Radix Rhapontici Seu Echinopsis**) is bitter, salty, and cold. It mainly treats skin heat, malign sores, flat abscesses, hemorrhoids, and damp impediment. It promotes lactation. Protracted taking may make the body light, boost the qi, sharpen the ears and eyes, prevent senility, and prolong life. Its other name is *Ye Lan* (Wild Orchid). It grows in mountains and valleys.

Qian Gen (**Radix Rubiae Cordifoliae**)[130] is bitter and cold. It mainly treats cold damp wind impediment and jaundice and supplements the center. It grows in mountains and valleys.

Xuan Hua (**Flos Calystegiae Sepii**)[131] is sweet and warm. It mainly boosts the qi and removes black patches from the face, thus rendering the facial complexion attractive. Its root [*i.e.*, Radix Calystegiae Sepii] mainly treats cold and heat and evil qi in the abdomen, and disinhibits urination. Protracted taking may make one free from hunger and the body light. Its other name is *Jin Gen Hua* (Sinewy Root Flower). Yet another name is *Jin Fei* (Boiling Gold). It grows in plains and swamps.

Bai Tu Huo (**Herba Cynanchi Caudati**) is bitter and balanced. It mainly treats bites by snakes and insects like bees, rabid dog bite, vegetable and meat toxins, *gu* toxins, and demonic influx. Its other name is *Bai Ge* (White Kudzu Vine). It grows in mountains and valleys.

---

[130] This medicinal is inclined to enter the constructive penetrating the blood. Therefore, it is able to move the blood to free the flow of the menses and disperse stasis. In addition, it is used to treat flooding and leaking, hematuria, knocks and falls, hemorrhoids and fistulas, sores, and nodes. Since impediment is due to the blood vessels being congested by wind, cold, and dampness and this medicinal is able to move the blood, impediment is one of its indications. Jaundice is produced from damp heat. It is, however, often complicated by blood amassment. Therefore, Rubia is also sometimes prescribed for jaundice.

[131] Although its name sounds like that of *Xuan Fu Hua* (Flos Inulae), these are two different medicinals.

Qing Xiang **(Herba Sesami Indici)**[132] is sweet and cold. It mainly treats evil qi in the five viscera and wind cold damp impediment. It boosts the qi, supplements the brain marrow, and fortifies the sinews and bones. Protracted taking may sharpen the ears and eyes, make one free from hunger, prevent senility, and increase longevity. It is the sprout of *Ju Sheng* (Sesame). It grows in rivers and valleys.

Dang Gui **(Radix Angelicae Sinensis)**[133] is sweet and warm. It is nontoxic, treating mainly cough and counterflow qi ascent, warm malaria with fever persisting within the skin, leaking causing infertility in females, various malign sores, and incised wounds. It can be [constantly] taken after being cooked. Its other name is *Gan Gui* (Dry Return). It grows in rivers and valleys.

---

[132] According to Tao Hong-jing, this medicinal is the leaves of sesame.

[133] *Dang Gui* (Radix Angelicae Sinensis) can be translated literally as "Expected to Be Back Home". It was said that if one missed one's relatives, one could send a dry piece of Dang Gui to the person, who, on receiving it, would come back. Dang Gui is a very important medicinal for blood troubles. It supplements the heart and harmonizes and moves the blood to disperse wind cold. It is all but indipensable for any women's disease. Ye Gui, a.k.a., Ye Tian-shi (1667-1746 CE), annotated this passage by saying:

> Once the blood becomes desiccated, liver wood will bring up heart fire to torment lung metal, thus giving rise to cough and counterflow qi ascent. Because Dang Gui enters the liver to nourish the blood and enters the heart to clear fire, it treats [cough and counterflow qi ascent]. Wind is attributed to the liver, while fire to the heart. Wind and fire are yang. Mere heat without cold is warm malaria which is due to wind and fire overwhelming the lungs. The lungs govern the skin and hair. Continual cold and heat in the skin reflects the lungs being subjected to wind and fire evils so they are not able to secure the skin and hair. Dang Gui enters the heart and liver. Once liver blood is made abundant, wind will be settled. Once heart blood is made abundant, fire will be extinguished and cold and heat in the skin and hair will be cured on its own. Leaking infertility is a result of blood desiccation. Since Dang Gui supplements the blood, this falls within its indications. All malign sores are ascribed to heart fire. When heart blood is made abundant, heart fire will be extinguished. As for incised wounds and loss of blood, since [Dang Gui] clears the heart and nourishes the blood, they are all its indications.

Herbs: Middle Class

Chi Jian (**Herba Gastrodiae Elatae**)[134] is acrid and warm. It mainly kills demonic and spiritual matters, *gu* toxins, and malign qi.[135] Protracted taking may boost the qi and [physical] force, help yin to grow, make one fat and strong and the body light, and lengthen life. Its other name is *Li Mu* (Parting Mother). Yet another name is *Gui Du You* (Ghost Post Governor). It grows in rivers and valleys.

---

[134] This medicinal is the herbal parts of Gastrodia, but nowadays we use the root (*i.e.*, Rhizoma Gastrodiae Elatae) which mainly treats various kinds of wind troubles and is very effective for head spinning with flowery (*i.e.*, blurred) vision.

[135] Malign qi means epidemic pestilential qi.

Mai Men Dong (Tuber Ophiopogonis Japonici)[136] is sweet and balanced. It mainly treats bound qi in the heart and abdomen, damaged center, overeating damage, [damaged] stomach, vessel network [or pulse] expiry, languor and emaciation, and shortness of breath. Protracted taking may make the body light, prevent senility, and make one free from hunger. It grows in rivers and valleys.

Juan Bai (Herba Selaginellae Involvensis) is acrid and balanced. It mainly treats evil qi in the five viscera and, in females, genital cold and heat and pain, concretions and conglomerations, blood block, and infertility. Protracted taking may make the body light and the facial complexion harmonious. Its other name is *Wan Sui* (Ten Thousand Years).[137] It grows in mountains and valleys.

---

[136] Ophiopogon is sweet and a little bitter in flavor and slightly cold of qi. As such, it is able to drain lung fire. Once lung fire is eliminated, the source of water will become clear and the heart will quiet down. Therefore, Ophiopogon is able to clear the heart, moisten the lungs to fortify yin, move water, and generate fluids. It follows that it is an important medicinal for resolving vexatious heat, dispersing phlegm, and suppressing cough due to yin vacuity. In addition, it treats wasting thirst, water swelling, lung wilting ejection of blood, and, in females, desiccated menses and breast milk stoppage. When stomach fire surges upward, it may give rise to vomiting. This kind of vomiting is also one of the indications of Ophiopogon.

In terms of the contraindications of this medicinal, Zou Shu (1790-1844 CE) said:

It cannot be used for lower burner repletion patterns unless there is vexatious heat in the palms and dryness of the lips and mouth. It cannot be used when the throat is uninhibited if qi ascent is caused by wind or phlegm rather than fire. [And] it cannot be used if vacuity emaciation with diminished qi is not complicated by qi counterflow and a desire to vomit but by diarrhea.

[137] Ten Thousand Years is a term used to express a wish of a long life or an epithet meaning eternal or evergreen. *Juan Bai* has a tough life. It can survive even if it has been uprooted and dried for many days. This is why it has acquired this name.

Rou Song Rong (**Herba Cistanchis Deserticolae**)[138] is salty. It mainly treats the five taxations and seven damages, supplements the center, eliminates cold and heat and pain in the penis, nourishes the five viscera, strengthens yin, and boosts the essence qi. In females, it makes pregnancy possible and [treats] concretions and conglomerations. Protracted taking may make the body light. It grows in mountains and valleys.

Ji Li Zi (**Semen Astragali Complanati**)[139] is bitter and warm. It mainly treats malign blood, breaks concretions and bindings, accumulations and gatherings, and [treats] throat impediment and difficult lactation. Protracted taking may promote the growth of the muscles and flesh, brighten the eyes, and make the body light. Its other name is *Pang Tong* (Free By-way). Yet another name is *Qu Ren* (Hamper to People). It is also called *Zhi Xing* (Stopping Walk), *Chai Yu* (Jackal Feather), and *Sheng Tui* (Upbearing Pushing).[140] It grows in plains and swamps.

---

[138] Nowadays, this medicinal is called *Rou Cong Rong*. It supplements life gate ministerial fire, moistens the five viscera, and boosts the essence and blood. Therefore, it treats taxation damage, cold pain in the lumbus and knees, flooding, vaginal discharge, and seminal emission. It is particularly good for infertility due to insufficiency and expiry of pure yang.

[139] Tribulus supplements the kidneys, drains the lungs, and dissipates liver wind. Therefore, it is able to treat vacuity taxation, lumbago, seminal emission, vaginal discharge, cough and counterflow, lung wilting, breast milk stoppage, and concretions and conglomerations. It boosts the essence and hence is able to brighten the eyes.

[140] This is so named because one of its main actions is to move and disperse blood so as to be able to hasten delivery.

43

Fang Feng **(Radix Ledebouriellae Divaricatae)**[141] is sweet and warm. It is nontoxic, treating mainly great wind head dizziness and headache, malign wind,[142] wind evil, blindness, wind moving around the whole body [causing] pain and impediment in the joints, and vexatious fullness. Protracted taking may make the body light. Its other name is *Tong Yun* (Bronze Rue). It grows in rivers and swamps.

Sha Shen **(Radix Glehniae Littoralis)**[143] is bitter and slightly cold. It is nontoxic, mainly treating blood accumulation and fright qi. It eliminates cold and heat, supplements the center, and boosts the lung qi. Protracted

---

[141] Zhang Zhi-cong, Ye Gui, and Xu Da-chun (1693-1771 CE) all attributed the indications of Ledebouriella listed in the text to its action of dispelling wind. Even blindness and vexatious fullness can be impugned to wind. As it is known, the liver opens into the eyes. When there is stirring of liver wind, the eyes will be impaired. Ledebouriella can track down such liver wind and, therefore, may cure blindness. In addition, though not mentioned in the text, it is a remedy for wind stroke with loss of the ability to speak because this disease is also due to wind. It should be noted that Ledebouriella can either promote or stop sweating depending upon what other medicinals it is combined with. Further, wind medicinals are usually simultaneously damp-dispelling medicinals. Conditions such as pain in the joints are typically due to wind combined with dampness. For that reason, this medicinal is also good for this type of problem.

[142] Malign wind implies a wind which is capable of causing a serious disease.

[143] Ginseng and Glehnia are both able to supplement the qi or, more specifically, the lung qi. Glehnia, however, is also able to supplement yin. Xu Da-chun said:

The lungs govern the qi. Therefore, medicinals for the lungs are mostly medicinals of overwhelming qi. However, medicinals of overwhelming qi are necessarily inclined to dry and those able to enrich the lungs are [mostly] sluggish and are unable to clear vacuity. Of these, only Glehnia is a medicinal which rectifies the blood in the lung qi division. It is white in color and light in weight. It dredges and is not drying; it is moistening but does not cause stagnation. When blood is held up in the lungs, nothing but this medicinal can clear it.

In a word, the action of this medicinal is mainly to boost the lung qi while simultaneously supplementing the spleen and kidneys.

taking brings benefit to people.[144] Its other name is *Zhi Mu* (Gratitude to Mother). It grows in rivers and valleys.

Xiong Qiong (Radix Ligustici Wallichii)[145] is acrid and warm. It is nontoxic, mainly treating wind stroke [with] wind entering the brain [causing] headache, cold impediment, hypertonicity of the sinews which are [sometimes] slack and [sometimes] tense, incised wounds, and, in females, blood block and infertility. It grows in rivers and valleys.

Mi Wu (Herba Ligustici Wallichii) is acrid and warm. It mainly treats cough and counterflow, settles fright qi, keeps off evils and malignancy, eliminates *gu* toxins and demonic influx, and removes the three [kinds of] worms. Protracted taking may enable one to communicate with spirits. Its other name is *Wei Wu* (Fine Weed). It grows in rivers and swamps.

---

[144] The Chinese word *li* is translated by Wiseman as "to disinhibit" when used in a Chinese medical sense, but nonmedically means to benefit.

[145] This medicinal is currently called *Chuan Xiong*. According to Zhu Zhen-heng, a.k.a., Zhu Dan-xi (1281-1358 CE), it is an able envoy leading to both yin and yang and both the blood and qi. It tends to ascend to open qi and blood depression. It is specifically effective for abdominal pain and headache. It can be used for headache related to all six channels requiring only that it be combined with other appropriate channel ushers. For example, to treat *tai yang* headache with aversion to wind and cold and a floating pulse, it should be prescribed with *Qiang Huo* (Radix Et Rhizoma Notopterygii) and *Man Jing Zi* (Fructus Viticis). For *yang ming* headache with pain along the route of the *yang ming* channel or spontaneous sweating, fever, no aversion to cold, and a floating, moderate, and long pulse, it should be combined with *Bai Zhi* (Radix Angelicae Dahuricae). If it is used in combination with *Chai Hu* (Radix Bupleuri), it treats *shao yang* headache with pain in the head along the route of the *shao yang* channel or headache characterized by alternating cold and heat and a bowstring pulse.

In addition, Ligusticum Wallichium is able to track wind, disperse stasis, and open depression. Therefore, it is often used in the treatment of menstrual disorders. It moistens liver dryness and supplements liver vacuity. This action makes it a good medicinal for all wind with shaking and dizzy vision, tearing, rib-side pain, and sinew hypertonicity. Moreover, because it harmonizes the blood and moves the qi, having access to both yin and yang, it is able to treat welling and flat abscesses and sores.

Xu Duan (**Radix Dypsaci**)[146] is bitter and slightly warm. It mainly treats cold damage, supplements insufficiency, [treats] incised wounds and welling abscesses, joins broken sinews and bones, and [resolves] difficult lactation in females. Protracted taking may boost the qi and [physical] force. Its other name is *Long Dou* (Dragon Bean). Another name is *Shu She* (Linking the Severed). It grows in mountains and valleys.

---

[146] In fact, there are three varieties of the plant—Lamium Album, Sonchus Asperis, and Dispsacus Japonicus. This medicinal mainly treats the foot *jue yin* and hand *shao yin*, and its actions include quickening, generating, and supplementing the blood. Ye Gui annotated this passage saying:

It mainly treats damaged center and supplements insufficiency, which means the supplementing of insufficiency of the liver channel. Incised wounds, welling abscesses, and [other] wounds are all troubles due to damaged blood. It is warm of qi and, therefore, boosts the blood. It is bitter in flavor and, therefore, enters the heart. On that account, [the above conditions] are indicated. In falls, the sinews may be severed and the bones broken. Because it quickens the blood and nourishes the channels, it may set fracture. When women's blood is insufficient, they will suffer from difficult lactation. Since its warm qi can move the blood, it naturally makes the breast milk abundant. The liver is the root of fatigue and exhaustion because it is the viscus which generates the qi and blood. The slightly warm qi [of this medicinal] accesses the *shao yang* qi. Therefore, it boosts the qi and [physical] force.

In modern clinical practice, this medicinal is also used to treat lumbago, blood dysentery, seminal emission, vaginal discharge, and fetal leakage or vaginal bleeding in pregnancy.

Yin Chen Hao (**Herba Artemisiae Capillaris**)[147] is bitter. It is nontoxic, treating mainly wind, damp, cold, and hot evil qi as well as bound heat jaundice. Protracted taking may make the body light, boost the qi, and slow aging. It grows on the hills and sides of Mount Tai.

Wu Wei (**Fructus Schisandrae Chinensis**)[148] is sour and warm. It mainly boosts the qi, [treating] cough and counterflow qi ascent, taxation damage, and languor and emaciation. It supplements insufficiency, fortifies yin, and boosts male's essence. It grows in mountains and valleys.

---

[147] Artemisa Capillaris is able to eliminate wind dampness and bound heat and disinhibit urination. It mainly treats heaven-current seasonal epidemics, headache, head spinning, eye pain, malaria, and concretions and conglomerations. It is specifically effective against jaundice. Generally speaking, jaundice is divided into two patterns, yin and yang. Yin jaundice refers to dull yellowing of the skin and eyes. It progresses slowly, and its symptoms and signs include the presence or absence of low fever, aversion to cold, no desire for food, fatigue and listlessness, sloppy stools, light yellow urine, a bland tongue body with white, glossy fur, and a bowstring and moderate or deep and slow pulse. Yang jaundice refers to bright yellowing of the body accompanied by fever, a bitter taste in the mouth, vexatious thirst, no desire for food, nausea, bound dry stools, yellow or reddish urine, and distention and fullness of the stomach duct. To treat yin jaundice, one should prescribe Artemisia Capillaris together with Ginger and Aconite, while yang jaundice requires Artemisia Capillaris in combination with Rhubarb and Gardenia.

[148] According to Wang Hao-gu's analysis, Schisandra constrains the lung qi and enriches kidney water. Therefore, it boosts the qi and generates fluids, fortifies yin and astringes the essence. It is often prescribed to stop vomiting and diarrhea, stabilize panting and coughing, and resolve wine toxins. Concerning the expression of fortifying yin, most scholars regard the term yin here as a generalized concept. However, Zou Shu had a different view. He said,""Chen Xiu-yuan (1753-1823 CE) alone is right when he explains it as treatment of impotence."

47

Qin Jiao (**Radix Gentianae Macrophyllae**)[149] is bitter and balanced. It mainly treats cold and heat, evil qi, and cold, damp, wind impediment with pain in the limb joints. It precipitates water and disinhibits urination. It grows in mountains and valleys.

Huang Qin (**Radix Scutellariae Baicalensis**)[150] is bitter and balanced. It mainly treats various [kinds of] heat, jaundice, intestinal afflux, diarrhea, and dysentery. It expels water, precipitates [*i.e.*, frees] blood block, and [treats] malign sores, flat abscesses, erosion [of flesh], and burns. Its other name is *Fu Chang* (Putrid Intestine). It grows in rivers and valleys.

---

[149] Gentiana Macrophylla disinhibits dampness, dissipates wind, removes heat from the stomach and intestines, and boosts the qi of the liver and gallbladder. When the *yang ming* suffers from heat, tidal fever and steaming bones arise. This is when Gentiana Macrophylla should be used. Because it nourishes the blood and nurtures the sinews, it treats hypertonicity and generalized pain. Since it is able to dissipate wind and eliminate cold, it is a remedy for wind cold damp impediment and toothache. Moreover, because it eliminates heat and disinhibits dampness, it is effective for jaundice.

[150] Scutellaria clears heart fire, drains lung fire, and treats upper burner heat, skin heat, and all other kinds of heat in both the interior and exterior. This is why the text says it mainly treats various (or all types of) heat jaundice, intestinal afflux and diarrhea. It also disinhibits the qi in the chest and disperses the phlegm above the diaphragm. When there is lung heat cough with copious phlegm and foul smell in the throat, it is the right medicinal to choose. Glomus fullness below the heart is due to heat. Therefore, Scutellaria is also prescribed for it. Besides, it is an important medicinal for women's diseases. Postpartum, it may nourish yin and abate yang, while during gestation, it may quiet the fetus. Loss of blood due to heat or postmenopausal recommencement of menstruation caused by blood heat also require Scutellaria. Finally, it may also be used as a remedy for dry bound stools, sore toxins, and other miscellaneous illnesses due to heat.

Shao Yao (**Radix Paeoniae Lactiflorae**)[151] is bitter. It mainly treats evil qi and abdominal pain, eliminates blood impediment, breaks hard gatherings and cold and heat mounting conglomeration, relieves pain, disinhibits urination, and boosts the qi. It grows in rivers and valleys.

---

[151] Peony is able to greatly drain liver fire. When wood is regulated, earth becomes quiet. Peony harmonizes the blood vessels, relaxes the center, relieves pain, contains the yin qi, constrains sweat, supplements taxation vacuity, and abates heat. Therefore, it treats spleen vacuity abdominal heat pain, heart glomus, rib-side pain, conglomeration, nosebleed, dry eyes, and all blood troubles.

Peony may produce other actions in addition to the above when it is used in combination with other appropriate medicinals. Together with Ginseng and Astragalus, it supplements the qi. When combined with Dang Gui and Rehmannia, it supplements the blood. Combining it with either Ligusticum Wallichium or Atractylodes enables it to supplement the spleen, while along with Licorice, it harmonizes yin to relieve abdominal pain. To relieve pain in the bone marrow, it is prescribed together with Tiger Bone, and, with the help of Rhinoceros Horn, it stops the hacking of blood and staunches nosebleed. If it is used together with Coptis, it cures dysentery and diarrhea.

There are two species of Peony, red and white. Red Peony (*i.e.*, Radix Rubrus Paeoniae Lactiflorae) more strongly drains liver fire, disperses malign blood, breaks hard accumulations, and relieves abdominal pain. White Peony (*i.e.*, Radix Albus Paeoniae Lactiflorae) more strongly constrains and supplements.

49

Gan Jiang (dry **Rhizoma Gingiberis**)[152] is acrid and warm. It mainly treats chest fullness, cough and counterflow qi ascent. It warms the center, stops bleeding, promotes perspiration, expels wind damp impediment, and [treats] intestinal afflux and dysentery. The uncooked is especially good. Protracted taking may remove foul smell and enable one to communicate with the spirit light. It grows in rivers and valleys.

---

[152] Apparently, the author is including both *Gan Jiang* (dry Ginger) and *Sheng Jiang* (uncooked Ginger) under this entry. Ginger's main actons are to warm the center and eliminate dampness. Secondarily, it may effuse and dissipate wind cold, stop vomiting, and disperse phlegm. In addition, it resolves worm and insect bite toxins and the toxicity of some medicinals.

When wind cold evils invade the chest, these may give rise to chest fullness. If these settle in the stomach and intestines, there may be glomus fullness, vomiting, pain in the abdomen, intestinal afflux, diarrhea, and dysentery. Wind cold in the blood is the cause of vomiting of blood and nosebleed, while wind cold in the sinews and bones is responsible for impediment. Ginger is indicated for all these troubles. Ginger is acrid and, as such, is able to dispel cold and promote sweating. Therefore, it also treats colds with headache and nasal congestion.

Together with Red Dates and Licorice, Ginger is able to regulate and supplement the spleen and stomach. The combination of Ginger and Peony warms the center and dissipates cold, a marvelous pair for pain in the middle and lower burner. When used together with Schisandra, Ginger treats cold cough. To generate blood and relieve pain, it is often used with Dang Gui and other medicinals. *Jiang Fu Tang* (Ginger & Aconite Decoction) is a miraculous formula for cold in the middle burner with the pulse bordering on expiry. If this formula is expanded by the addition of Licorice, it may salvage and restore expired yang. Then it is called *Si Ni Tang* (Four Counterflows Decoction).

It is said that Confucius never ate a meal without Ginger. Maybe he did this to rid his food of any bad smell so as to increase his appetite. This may be what is meant by the phrase "removing foul smell" in the text. However, in some versions, this phrase is, "removes foul smell above the diaphragm in the chest."

Dry and uncooked Ginger have similar actions. Uncooked Ginger is comparatively less warming but stronger for effusing and dissipating. Blast-fried Ginger (*Pao Jiang*) is also frequently used. It is less acrid and is able to treat lung wilt, postpartum blood vacuity, hot body with internal cold, vomiting of blood, and nosebleed.

Gao Ben (**Radix Et Rhizoma Ligustici Chinensis**)[153] is acrid and slightly warm. It mainly treats mounting conglomeration and genital cold in females, swelling and pain, and abdominal urgency. It eliminates wind headache, promotes the growth of muscles and skin, and renders the facial complexion attractive. Its other name is *Gui Qing* (Ghost Minister). Another name is *Di Xin* (New Earth). It grows in mountains and valleys.

Ma Huang (**Herba Ephedrae**)[154] is bitter and warm. It is nontoxic, treating mainly wind stroke cold damage, headache, and warm malaria. It effuses the exterior [through] sweating, eliminates evil heat qi, suppresses cough and counterflow qi ascent, eliminates cold and heat, and breaks

---

[153] The main action of Ligusticum Chinensis is to eliminate wind, cold, and dampness. When combined with Ligusticum Wallichium, Cimicifuga, Ledebouriella, and Bupleurum, Ligusticum Chinensis is an effective medicinal for treating pain in the top of the head. If wind settles in the stomach giving rise to diarrhea or if cold dampness settles in the abdomen causing acute pain, Ligusticum Chinensis can also be prescribed.

[154] Tao Hong-jing (452-536 CE) said, "Ephedra is the first choice in treating cold damage and resolving the muscles." Whenever any surplus evil of the six excesses (*i.e.*, cold, summerheat, dampness, etc.) settles in the yang division in the skin and hair shutting the interstices and bringing the constructive and defensive to a stop —an exterior repletion pattern—Ephedra never fails to open and free the interstices to drive out the evil through sweating. For instance, a single dose of Ephedra, Cinnamon Twig, Armeniaca, and Licorice may effect the cure of a *tai yang* pattern of wind cold in the exterior with pain and stiffness in the head and back of the neck, fever, generalized joint pain, a floating, tight pulse, absence of sweating, chest fullness, and panting. These medicinals make up the formula called *Ma Huang Tang* (Ephedra Decoction). In the *Yi Zong Jin Jian (Golden Mirror of Ancestral Medicine)* edited by Wu Qian, there is a passage dealing with *Ma Huang Tang* which says:

> People say Ephedra is specifically able to effuse the exterior but cannot treat other diseases. They do not know this decoction. After being combined with *Gui Zhi Tang* (Cinnamon Twig Decoction), it is called *Ma Gui Ge Ban Tang* (Half Ephedra & Half Cinnamon Decoction). This can be used to treat persisting cold and heat in the *tai yang* pattern...

This says that Ephedra is also able to treat an interior condition through effusing the exterior. Therefore, it may be used in treatment of wind stroke, jaundice, etc.

51

concretions and hardness, accumulations and gatherings. Its other name is *Long Sha* (Dragon Sand). It grows in rivers and valleys.

Ge Gen **(Radix Puerariae)**[155] is sweet and balanced. It mainly treats wasting thirst, generalized great fever, retching and vomiting, and various [kinds of] impediment. It lifts yin qi and resolves various [kinds of] toxins. *Ge Gu* (Semen Puerariae) mainly treats more than 10 year-old dysentery. Its other name is *Ji Qi Gen* (Chicken-like Root). It grows in rivers and valleys.

Zhi Mu **(Rhizoma Anemarrhenae Asphodeloidis)**[156] is bitter and cold. It is nontoxic, mainly treating wasting thirst and heat in the center. It eliminates evil qi [in the treatment of] puffy swelling of the limbs, precipitates water, supplements insufficiency, and boosts the qi. Its other name is *Chi Mu* (Ant Egg Mother). Another name is *Lian Mu* (Linking Mother). It is also called *Ye Liao* (Wild Water Weed), *Di Shen* (Earth Ginseng), *Shui Shen* (Water Ginseng), *Shui Jun* (Water Dredger), *Huo Mu* (Goods Matrix), and *Ti Mu* (Cicada Mother). It grows in rivers and valleys.

---

[155] The actions of Pueraria are to lift fluids from the stomach to moisten the lungs and dissipate exterior evils to resolve the muscles. It mainly treats wasting thirst, intense fever, headache, retching and vomiting, and wine toxins. For this last indication, the flower (Flos Puerariae) is better than the root. In addition, it is a good medicinal for spleen vacuity thirst.

[156] Anemarrhena drains fire through disinhibiting urination. Therefore, it treats wasting thirst, vexatious fever, alternating cold and heat, etc. It is a well known yin-boosting medicinal, but it should not be taken as a yin-supplementing one because taking too much of it may actually damage yin.

Bei Mu (**Bulbus Fritillariae**)[157] is acrid and balanced. It mainly treats cold damage, vexatious fever, dribbling, evil qi, mounting conglomeration, throat impediment, difficult lactation, incised wounds, and wind tetany. Its other name is *Kong Cao* (Hollow Weed).

---

[157] Fritillaria opens depression and resolves binding, downbears heart fire and moistens the lungs, clears phlegm and stops cough. It treats vexatious fever, ejection and hacking of blood, lung wilting, lung abscess, goiters, fistulas, malign sores, strangury, difficult delivery, and retention of the placenta. However, its main indications are the treatment of lung troubles.

Zou Shu gave an annotation to this passage which is focused on the analysis of phlegm rheum. He said:

When phlegm drool gathers in the heart and chest, [heart] yin will be unable to descend. In consequence, cold damage will have the signs of vexatious fever and dribbling [urination]. If phlegm drool gathers in the throat, the evil qi will make it difficult for yang [qi] to ascend. As a result, the illness of throat impediment arises. Because [phlegm drool] makes it impossible to transform and return blood to the *chong* [vessel], difficult lactation arises. Mounting conglomeration is due to phlegm drool obstructing the *ren* vessel in the heart and chest. Wind tetany is produced by phlegm drool gathering in the heart and chest to deprive the governing vessel of yin [nourishment] for irrigation. Incised wounds seem to have nothing to do with phlegm drool. However, profuse bleeding may cause shortage of yin which cannot be recruited. Then the qi gathers and fails to transform and, instead, becomes depressed and bound in the heart and chest. Thus phlegm drool is produced. The principal medicinal [for these disorders] is Fritillaria which may quickly initiate transformation...

53

Gua Lou (**Fructus Trichosanthis Kirlowii**)[158] is bitter and cold. It mainly treats wasting thirst, generalized fever, vexatious fullness, and great heat. It supplements vacuity, quiets the center, and mends expiry and damage. Its other name is *Di Lou* (Earth Building). It grows in rivers and valleys as well as shady places in the mountains.

---

[158] Trichosanthes clears upper burner fire, moistens the lungs, flushes phlegm, and disinhibits the throat. As such, it is an ideal medicinal for cough and a miraculous one for thirst. It also treats abscesses, swellings, sores, and various toxins. In the text, it is said to be bitter, but actually it is bitter and sweet. Therefore, unlike purely bitter medicinals, it does not damage the stomach.

Trichosanthes and Pinellia are both able to treat phlegm and cough, but they work in different ways. Zhang Zhi-cong said:

Pinellia lifts the yin qi from outside the vessels, making it meet the *yang ming* above so that it turns [the qi] into dry fire and earth. Trichosanthes Root lifts yin fluids from inside the vessels, making it meet the *tian gui* [*i.e.,* kidney water] so as to enrich dry metal. In the various formulas in the *Shan Han* (*[Treatsie on] Cold Damage*) and the *Jin Gui* (*[Essentials from] the Golden Cabinet*), Pinellia is used to assist the *yang ming* qi. If there is thirst due to excessive dryness and heat, Pinellia should be replaced by *Hua Fen* (Radix Trichosanthis Kirlowii) in order to enrich [water]...

54

Dan Shen **(Radix Salviae Miltiorrhizae)**[159] is bitter and slightly cold. It is nontoxic, treating mainly evil qi in the heart and abdomen, continual gurgling of the intestines like water running, cold and heat, and gatherings and accumulations. It breaks concretions and eliminates conglomerations, relieves vexatious fullness, and boosts the qi. Its other name is *Que Chan Cao* (Cicada-deterring Weed). It grows in mountains and valleys.

Xuan Shen **(Radix Scrophulariae Ningpoensis)**[160] is bitter and slightly cold. It is nontoxic, treating mainly cold and heat accumulations and gatherings in the abdomen and, in females, postpartum illnesses and illnesses related to breast-feeding. It supplements the kidney qi and

---

[159] Salvia breaks blood stasis, nourishes the blood, and engenders new blood. It is an important medicinal for women's diseases. It regulates menstruation, quiets the fetus, precipitates the dead fetus, and treats flooding, vaginal discharge, and concretions and conglomerations. It is also marvelous for quieting the spirit, stabilizing the will, and freeing the flow of the blood vessels. Continual rumbling of the intestines, as Zou Shu said, was due to:

...obstructed heart qi being unable to go up or down. Therefore, it must descend into the intestines.

Because Salvia is able to supplement the heart qi and eliminate evil qi, rumbling of the intestines is also one of its indications. However, if rumbling intestines, concretions and conglomerations, etc. are not caused by evil qi in the heart and chest, this medicinal is ineffective. In modern clinical practice, Salvia is also used to treat weak feet, painful impediment, and malign stroke as well as to expel pus and relieve pain.

[160] Scrophularia invigorates water to abate fire and, therefore, is a good medicinal for dissipating rootless fire. It is used to treat languor and insomnia, confused spirit, vexatious thirst, throat impediment, sore throat, urinary and fecal stoppage, yang toxin macular eruption, steaming bones, tidal fever, scrofulas, welling and flat abscesses, and mouse scrofulas. Chen Nian-zu, a.k.a. Chen Xiu-yuan (1753-1823 CE) said:

In postpartum blood desertion, yin is exhausted and fire has nothing to restrain it. If this is treated with cold and cool [medicinals], there is fear of damaging the center. If drastically supplementing [medicinals] are added, there is a fear of [these medicinals] repelling each other. Luckily, Scrophularia is able to clear and slightly supplement, so it is an important medicinal for postpartum disorders.

brightens the eyes. Its other name is *Chong Tai* (Multi-storey Platform). It grows in rivers and valleys.

Ku Shen (**Radix Sophorae Flavescentis**)[161] is bitter and cold. It mainly treats bound qi in the heart and abdomen, concretions and conglomerations, accumulations and gatherings, jaundice, and dribbling after voiding. It expels water, eliminates welling abscesses and swellings, supplements the center, brightens the eyes, and stops tearing. Its other name is *Shui Huai* (Water Scholartree). Another name is *Ku Shi* (Bitter Aniseed). It grows in mountains and valleys as well as fields.

Gou Ji (**Rhizoma Cibotii Barometsis**)[162] is bitter and balanced. It mainly treats rigidity of the upper and lower back, slack and tense joints, generalized impediment, and cold damp knee pain. It benefits old people very much. Its other name is *Bai Zhi* (Hundred Branches). It grows in rivers and valleys.

Bei Xie (**Rhizoma Dioscoreae Hypoglaucae**)[163] is bitter and balanced. It mainly treats pain and rigidity of the upper and lower back and the joints, wind cold damp limb joint and generalized impediment, intractable malign sores, and heat qi. It grows in mountains and valleys.

---

[161] Sophora Flavescens drains fire and dries dampness, supplements yin and boosts the essence, nourishes the liver and gallbladder, disinhibits the nine orifices, and quenches thirst. It treats dysentery, jaundice, reddish urine, malign sores, and invisible worm sores (*i.e.*, vaginal ulcers). In the text, this medicinal is said to be able to supplement the center. This is because it is bitter in flavor and, as such, is able to dry dampness. The spleen is averse to dampness. When dampness is removed, the spleen is fortified.

[162] This medicinal supplements the liver and kidneys. Once these viscera are made strong, the sinews and bones will also become strong.

[163] Dioscorea Hypoglauca is specifically capable of expelling wind dampness and normalizing urination. When wind dampness is removed, the sinews and bones will become normal and strong. Therefore, it is a good medicinal for generalized impediment and rigidity and pain of the back.

Tong Cao (**Caulis Akebiae**)[164] is acrid and balanced. It mainly removes malign worms, eliminates cold and heat of the spleen and stomach, and disinhibits and frees the nine orifices, blood vessels, and joints. It may improve memory. Its other name is *Fu Zhi* (Appending Branch). It grows in mountains and valleys.

Qu Mai (**Herba Dianthi**)[165] is bitter and cold. It mainly treats block and repulsion and various [kinds of] dribbling, binding, and urinary stoppage. It removes thorns, opens welling abscesses and swellings, brightens the eyes, eliminates [eye] screen, breaks the placenta and drops the fetus,[166] and precipitates blocked [*i.e.*, dead] blood. Its other name is *Ju Ju Mai* (Giant Wheat). It grows in rivers and valleys.

Bai Jiang (**Herba Patriniae Heterophyllae Cum Radice**) is bitter and balanced. It mainly treats fulminant heat, burns, red qi [*i.e.*, blood diseases], scabs, flat abscesses, hemorrhoids, horse saddle [bruises], and heat qi. Its other name is *Lu Chang* (Deer Intestine). It grows in rivers and valleys.

---

[164] One should note that, before the Song dynasty, what is now called *Mu Tong* was called *Tong Cao* and vice versa. Akebia downbears heart fire, clears lung heat, abducts damp heat out through urination, and disinhibits the blood vessels and joints. It is an important medicinal for disinhibiting urination, promoting lactation, and freeing the flow of the channels. Yang Shi-ying, a.k.a. Yang Ren-zhai, a prolific medical writer of the Song dynasty, wrote:

> Generalized dull heat and pain, hypertonicity, and cold feet are all due to hidden heat damaging the blood and require Akebia to free the heart orifices. When the channel and vessel networks enjoy free circulation, these diseases will be eliminated.

[165] This medicinal is good at disinhibiting. It downbears fire and, therefore, is a miraculous medicinal for strangury.

[166] This implies that this medicinal is able to precipitate a dead fetus.

Bai Zhi (**Radix Angelicae Dahuricae**)[167] is acrid and warm. It mainly treats leaking, red and white [vaginal discharge], blood block, and swollen genitals in females, and cold and heat, head wind, and [wind] invading the eyes causing tearing. It promotes the growth of the muscles and skin and moistens and makes [the skin] shiny. It can be used to make a face cream. Its other name is *Fang Xiang* (Fragrance). It grows in rivers and valleys.

Du Ruo (**Radix Polliae Japonicae**) is acrid and slightly warm. It mainly treats the chest and rib-side region. It precipitates counterflow qi, warms the center, and [is good for] wind invading the brain door,[168] swollen head and headache, copious snivel, and tearing. Protracted taking may boost the essence, brighten the eyes, and make the body light. Its other name is *Du Heng* (Horizontal Peartree). It grows in rivers and swamps.

Zi Cao (**Radix Lithospermi Seu Arnebiae**)[169] is bitter and cold. It mainly treats evil qi in the heart and abdomen and the five [kinds of] jaundice. It supplements the center, boosts the qi, disinhibits the nine orifices, and frees the flow of the water passageways. Its other name is *Zi Dan* (Purple Elixir). Another name is *Zi Ao* (Purple Pigment). It is also called *Di Xue* (Earth Blood). It grows in mountains and valleys.

---

[167] Angelica Dahurica dissipates wind, dispels dampness, frees the orifices, and promotes perspiration. It is often used as an usher to the hand and foot *yang ming* and *jue yin* and hand *tai yin*. The *yang ming* travels the face and head. When there is headache and blurred vision, one may prescribe Angelica Dahurica with Ligusticum Wallichium. If there is supraorbital pain, it may be combined with Notopterygium and Scutellaria. In addition, Angelica Dahurica treats toothache, deep-source nasal congestion, itching of the eyes, and tearing, and it is often used to treat wind stroke (either bowel or visceral stroke), leaking, blood block, and genital swelling. These disorders are usually due to wind cold complicated by damp heat.

[168] This refers to the area around the point *Nao Hu* (GV 17). When wind enters the brain through the brain door (*nao hu*), it may give rise to pain at the vertex and, in extreme cases, to retching and vomiting and dizziness.

[169] Lithospermum cools and quickens the blood, disinhibits the nine orifices, and frees urination and defecation. Therefore, it is able to treat heart and abdominal evil qi, water swelling, and the five categories of jaundice (*i.e.*, grain, wine, and sex jaundice, yellowing, and yellow sweating).

Zi Wan (**Radix Asteris Tatarici**)[170] is bitter and warm. It mainly treats cough and counterflow qi ascent and cold and heat bound qi in the chest. It eliminates *gu* toxins and crippling wilt and quiets the five viscera. It grows in mountains and valleys.

Bai Xian (**Cortex Radicis Dictamni Dasycarpi**)[171] is bitter and cold. It mainly treats head wind, jaundice, cough and counterflow, dribbling, genital swelling and pain in females, damp impediment, dead muscles, and inability to bend or stretch [the joints] and to walk or stand. It grows in rivers and valleys.

Wei Xin (**Herba Gnaphalii Affineae**)[172] is bitter and balanced. It mainly treats wind damp impediment, joint-running pain, fright epilepsy, protrusion of the tongue, palpitation qi, bandit wind, mouse fistulas, and welling abscesses and swellings. Its other name is *Mi Xin* (Elk Bite). It grows in rivers and swamps.

---

[170] Aster supplements vacuity and regulates the center, treating cold and heat bound qi, coughing and ejection of pus and blood. It is a miraculous medicinal for vacuity heat and vacuity taxation.

[171] This medicinal is dry in nature and, as such, is able to penetrate and break block. Therefore, it is used to disinhibit the joints, free the nine orifices, and move the water passageways. In modern times, it is used to treat jaundice, wind impediment, weak sinews and bones, heat sores, scabs, brittle hair, and hair loss. Genital swelling in females is usually due to accumulation of damp heat. Because Dictamnus can dry dampness, it is also prescribed to treat such troubles as well.

[172] This medicinal is hard to identify. Many herbs have been suggested for it. One possibility is Herba Salriae Nippomicae.

Bai Wei (**Radix Cynanchi Baiwei**)[173] is bitter and balanced. It mainly treats sudden wind stroke, generalized fever, limb fullness [*i.e.*, distention], sudden inability to recognize people, manic and confusing evil qi, cold and heat, aching pain, and distressing warm malaria which attacks at regular intervals. It grows in rivers and valleys.

Xi Er Shi (**Fructus Xanthii Sibirici**)[174] is sweet and warm. It mainly treats wind and cold headache, wind damp generalized impediment, hypertonicity and pain of the limbs, and malign flesh and dead muscles. Protracted taking may boost the qi, sharpen the ears and eyes, strengthen the will, and make the body light. Its other name is *Hu Xi* (Nomad's Earring). Another name is *Di Kui* (Earth Big Flower). It grows in rivers and valleys.

Mao Gen (**Rhizoma Imperatae Cylindricae**)[175] is sweet and cold. It mainly treats taxation damage, vacuity, and languor, supplements the center, boosts the qi, eliminates blood stasis, blood block, cold and heat, and disinhibits urination. The sprout [*i.e.*, young Herba Imperatae Cylindricae]

---

[173] Cynanchum is a medicinal for the *yang ming*, the *ren* and *chong* vessels. It boosts the yin qi and precipitates water qi so as to treat yin vacuity and effulgent fire, wind phlegm congestion causing generalized fever, limb distention, and inability to recognize people. Cynanchum is able to drain heat. Therefore, when heat is cleared, wind will die down, and when phlegm is cleared, soberness will be regained. In addition, this medicinal also treats evil qi warm malaria with alternating fever and chills, and generalized aching pain and, in females, gestational and postpartum enuresis. These troubles are all due to blood heat. So-called sudden wind stroke is also called *xue jue* (blood inversal) or *yu mao* (depression faintness). It is characterized by copious sweating, shortage of blood, qi congested so as to be at a stop, and sudden loss of consciousness or confused mind. To treat this, Cynanchum is prescribed together with Peony.

[174] The current name of this medicinal is *Cang Er*.

[175] Imperata supplements the center, drains fire, disinhibits urination, disperses blood stasis, and stops various types of bleeding. As a matter of fact, it is a remedy for any illnesses related to the blood, such as taxation detriment ejection of blood, nosebleeding, flooding, stagnant blood from falls and knocks, and blood block with cold and heat in females. It also treats hiccough, lung heat rapid panting, and internal heat vexatious thirst.

mainly precipitates water. Its other name is *Lan Gen* (Orchid Root). Another name is *Ru Gen* (Linked Root). It grows in mountains and valleys.

Suan Jiang (**Herba Physalis Alkekengi**) is sour and balanced. It mainly treats heat and vexatious fullness, settles the will, boosts the qi, and disinhibits the water passageways. In case of difficult delivery, swallowing its seed [*i.e.*, Semen Physalis Alkekengi] may effect instant delivery. Its other name is *Cu Jiang* (Paste Vinegar). It grows in rivers and swamps.

Yin Yang Huo (**Herba Epimedii**)[176] is acrid and cold. It mainly treats impotence, expiry and damage, and pain in the penis. It disinhibits urination, boosts the qi and [physical] force, and strengthens the will. Its other name is *Gang Qian* (Staunch Front). It grows in mountains and valleys.

Li Shi (**Semen Iridis Pallasii**)[177] is sweet and balanced. It mainly treats cold and heat in the skin, heat qi in the stomach, and wind, cold, damp impediment. It fortifies the sinews and bones and makes one desire food. Protracted taking may make the body light. Its flowers and leaves [*i.e.*, Flos Et Folium Iridis Pallasii] are able to remove white worms [*i.e.*, pinworms]. Its other name is *Ju Cao* (Sharp Weed). Another name is *San Jian* (Three Hard). It is also called *Shi Shou* (Pig Head). It grows in rivers and valleys.

---

[176] Epimedium boosts the essence and qi, fortifies the sinews and bones, and disinhibits urination. It treats paraplegia and insensitivity of the skin. It is an important medicinal for impotence due to expiry of yang in males and infertility due to expiry of yin in females. The phrase expiry and damage means expiry of the network vessels which are the passageways for yin essence and yang qi. If these expire or are damaged, impotence and infertility will arise.

[177] The name of this medicinal does not agree with the description of its indications. Therefore, its identity is questionable.

Kuan Dong (Flos Tussilaginis Farfarae)[178] is acrid and warm. It mainly treats cough and counterflow qi ascent, frequent panting, throat impediment, various [kinds of] fright epilepsy, and cold and heat evil qi. Its other name is *Tuo Wu* (Stone Bag). Another name is *Ke Dong* (Frozen Stalk). It is also called *Hu Xu* (Tiger Beard) and *Tu Yuan* (Hare Nest). It grows in mountains and valleys.

Fang Ji (Radix Stephaniae Tetrandrae)[179] is acrid and balanced. It mainly treats wind and cold, warm malaria, heat qi, and various [kinds of] epilepsy. It eliminates evils [through] disinhibiting urination and defecation. Its other name is *Jie Li* (Wheel Spoke). It grows in rivers and valleys.

Nu Wan (Radix Asteris Fastigiati)[180] is acrid and warm. It mainly treats continual wind cold, sudden turmoil [*i.e.*, choleraic disease], diarrhea and dysentery, rumbling in the intestines which goes up and down and is not fixed in place, fright epilepsy, and hundreds of diseases with cold and heat. It grows in rivers and valleys.

---

[178] Tussilago is an important medicinal for warming the lungs and suppressing cough. It is used to treat cough, panting, throat impediment, lung abscess, lung wilting, and coughing and ejecting of blood. However it is good only for cold dampness. If these conditions are due to fire heat tormenting the lungs, it is no longer the appropriate medicinal.

[179] There are two species of *Fang Ji*—*Mu Fang Ji* (Cocculus Trilobi) and *Han Fang Ji* (Stephania Tetrandra). In olden times, *Mu Fang Ji* and *Han Fang Ji* were distinguished in different ways. In some old classics, they were regarded even as the same plant, and, according to this approach, the distinction between the two was simply that *Mu Fang Ji* was the root, while *Han Fang Ji* was the aerial plant. In modern prescriptions, no differentiation is made between them.

This medicinal is specific for the foot *tai yang* channel but it is able to penetrate all 12 channels. It frees the interstices, disinhibits the nine orifices, and drains damp heat from the blood division of the lower burner. Therefore, it treats water swelling, generalized swelling (*i.e.*, edema), wind water with panting and coughing, and cold damp feet leading eventually to swollen feet.

[180] *Nu Wan* (Aster Fastigiatus) and *Zi Wan* (Aster Tataris) belong to the same species. Nowadays, only Aster Tataris is used in Chinese medicine.

Ze Lan **(Herba Lycopi Lucidi)**[181] is sour. It is nontoxic, treating mainly breast-feeding women,[182] nosebleed, illnesses following wind stroke, enlarged abdomen with water swelling, puffy swelling of the trunk, face, and limbs, water inside the bone joints, incised wounds, welling abscesses and swellings, sores, and suppuration. Its other name is *Hu Lan* (Tiger Orchid). Another name is *Long Zao* (Dragon Date). It grows by the side of pools.

Di Yu **(Radix Sanguisorbae Officinalis)**[183] is bitter and slightly cold. It mainly treats women with milk stagnation pain, the seven damages, and vaginal discharge disease. It relieves pain, eliminates malign flesh, stops sweating, and heals incised wounds. It grows in mountains and valleys.

Wang Sun **(Rhizoma Paridis Tetraphyllae)** is bitter and balanced. It is nontoxic, treating mainly evil qi in the five viscera, cold damp impediment, aching pain in the limbs, and cold pain in the knees. It grows in rivers and valleys.

Jiao Chuang **(Herba Justiciae Procumbensis)** is salty and cold. It mainly treats pain in the lumbar spine which is unable to touch the bed and where there is difficulty bending forward and back. It eliminates heat and can be used to make bathwater.

---

[181] Lycopus should be acrid and bitter, and a little warm rather than sour as in the text. This medicinal frees the nine orifices, disinhibits the joints, boosts the qi, and moves the blood. Because it is able to supplement without causing stagnation and move the blood and qi in a moderate way, it is an ideal medicinal for the treatment of taxation detriment, abdominal pain, lumbago, and, in females, various gestational and postpartum diseases. Its other indications, such as incised wounds, concretions, and water, are all based on its actions of breaking the blood and dispersing stasis.

[182] As a matter of fact, this medicinal is not limited to the treatment of breast-feeding women. It is a remedy for various diseases in females, for example, conditions related to pregnancy and birthing, abdominal pain, lumbago, and taxation.

[183] Sanguisorba enters the foot *jue yin* and blood division of the lower burner. It eliminates blood heat and stops bleeding. Therefore, it is a good medicinal for blood dysentery, vaginal discharge, incised wounds, etc.

Ma Xian Hao (Herba Pedicularis Resupinatae) is acrid and balanced. It mainly treats cold and heat, demonic influx, wind stroke, damp impediment, and, in females, vaginal discharge disease and infertility. Its other name is *Ma Shi Hao* (Horse Droppings Tall Weed). It grows in rivers and swamps.

Shu Yang Quan (Herba Solani Lyrati) is bitter and slightly cold. It mainly treats baldness, malign sores, heat qi, scabs, and lichen worms. It cures tooth decay. It grows in rivers and valleys.

Ji Xue Cao (Herba Hydrocotyle Asiaticae) is bitter and cold. It mainly treats great heat, malign sores, welling and flat abscesses, wet, spreading sores, red *biao*,[184] reddening of the skin, and generalized fever. It grows in rivers and valleys.

Yuan Yi (Herba Musci)[185] is sour. It is nontoxic, treating mainly jaundice, heart vexation, cough and counterflow, blood and qi, and fulminant heat in the stomach and intestines. It stops incised wounds.[186] Protracted taking may supplement the center, boost the qi, promote growth of the muscles, and render the facial complexion good. Its other name is *Xi Xie* (Past Evil). Another name is *Wu Jiu* (Black Leek). It is also called *Yuan Ying* (Ying on the Wall), *Tian Jiu* (Celestial Leek), and *Shu Jiu* (Mouse Leek). It grows on the north side of old walls or over the roofs of old houses.

---

[184] *Biao* refers to acute, infectious, suppurating sores on the fingers, toes, palms of the hands, and soles of the feet.

[185] This refers to a group of species of moss growing over old walls and the roofs of old houses.

[186] According to our reading, this sentence means that this medicinal is able to heal incised wounds. However, some scholars interpret the words *jin chuang nei sai* as a single term meaning lockjaw.

Shui Ping (**Herba Lemnae Seu Spirodelae**)[187] is acrid and cold. It mainly treats fulminant heat and generalized itching, precipitates water qi, [helps] get over wine, promotes the growth of the beard and [head] hair, and quenches wasting thirst. Protracted taking may make the body light. Its other name is *Shui Hua* (Water Flower). It grows in pools and swamps.

Hai Zao (**Herba Sargassii**) is bitter and cold. It mainly treats goiters and tumors and nodes in the neck. It breaks and disperses bound qi, welling abscesses and swellings, and concretions and accumulation hardness qi. [It stops] abdominal rumbling going up and down and precipitates the 12 [kinds of] water swelling.[188] Its other name is *Luo Shou* (Fallen Head). It grows in pools and swamps.

Jie Geng (**Radix Platycodi Grandiflori**)[189] is bitter. It is nontoxic, treating mainly chest and rib-side pain as if stabbed by a knife, abdominal fullness, continual intestinal rumbling, and fright and fear palpitation qi. It grows in mountains and valleys.

---

[187] This medicinal is good for promoting sweating, even better than Ephedra. It is indicated for addictive papules, heat sores, and wind warm diseases that are due to wind.

[188] Water swelling can be classified in a number of different ways. The translator has not been able to identify a specific set of 12.

[189] Platycodon drains lung heat, lifts the blood and qi, clears the head, eyes, and throat, rectifies the qi in the chest, nourishes the blood, and expels pus. For that reason, it is an important medicinal for lung abscesses, phlegm panting, cough, nasal congestion, red eyes, throat impediment and sore throat, toothache, and mouth sores. In addition, because it is able to disperse fire depression in the lower burner, it treats dysentery, abdominal pain, and rumbling intestines. Zhang Yuan-su likened Platycodon to a boat which is able to carry various bitter-flavored downbearing medicinals to break glomus, chest fullness, chest binding, etc. Chest binding is a syndrome comprised of distention, pain, and hardness below the heart usually accompanied by fever.

Xuan Fu Hua (**Flos Inulae**)[190] is salty and warm. It mainly treats bound qi, rib-side fullness, and fright palpitations, removes water, eliminates cold and heat in the five viscera, supplements the center, and downbears the qi. Its other name is *Jin Fei Cao* (Boiling Gold Weed). Another name is *Sheng Zhan* (Profound Clearness). It grows in rivers and valleys.

She Quan (**Herba Potentillae Kleinianae**) is bitter and slightly cold. It mainly treats fright epilepsy, cold and heat, and evil qi. It eliminates heat and [is good for] incised wounds, flat abscesses, hemorrhoids, mouse fistulas, malign sores, and head sores. Its other name is *She Xin* (Snakebite). It grows in mountains and valleys.

Jia Su (**Herba Schizonepetae Tenuifoliae**)[191] is acrid and warm. It mainly treats cold and heat, mouse fistulas, scrofulas, and sores. It breaks bound and gathered qi, precipitates blood stasis, and eliminates damp impediment. Its other name is *Shu Ming* (Mouse Water Chestnut). It grows in rivers and swamps.

---

[190] There is a saying that, "All the hundreds of flowers downbear except for Inula which upbears." It precipitates the qi and moves water and, therefore, is able to treat phlegm glomus, water swelling due to the large intestine, head wind, and belching.

[191] The current name of this medicinal is *Jing Jie*. It promotes sweating, dissipates wind, resolves binding, clears the head and eyes, disinhibits the blood vessels, stops vomiting, stops nosebleeding, disperses food, and recuperates from the effects of alcohol. It is a miraculous medicinal for wind and blood troubles and sores. In addition, it is effective for postpartum blood faintness.

Herbs: Inferior Class

Ying Shi (**Semen Rosae Multiflorae**)[192] is sour and warm. It mainly treats welling and flat abscesses, malign sores, flesh binding, sprained sinews, putrefying sores, heat qi, and intractable genital erosion. It [also] disinhibits the joints. Its other name is *Qiang Wei* (Wall Rose). Another name is *Qiang Ma* (Wall Flax). It is also called *Niu Ji* (Cow Bramble). It grows in rivers and valleys.

Mu Dan (**Cortex Radicis Moutan**)[193] is acrid and cold. It mainly treats cold and heat, wind stroke, tugging and slackening tetany, and fright epilepsy evil qi. It eliminates concretions, hardness, and blood stasis lodged in the stomach and intestines, quiets the five viscera, and cures abscesses and sores. Its other name is *Lu Jiu* (Deer Leek). Another name is *Shu Gu* (Mouse Aunt). It grows in mountains and valleys.

---

[192] Semen Rosae Multiflorae is used to treat thorns in the flesh, fish bones stuck in the throat, etc. The translator suspects that the indications explained in the text are those of Radix Rosae Multiflorae.

[193] Moutan is particularly able to drain fire hidden in the blood. It is often used to harmonize, cool, and generate the blood, to break accumulated blood, and to free the flow of the channels. It is an important medicinal for treating blood ejection and nosebleeding. It is also effective for steaming bones. Zhang Yuan-su said, "Moutan treats sweat-absent steaming bones, while Lycium Root Bark treats steaming bones with perspiration." In this passage, Moutan is said to treat tugging and slackening, tetany, and fright epilepsy evil qi. The reason is that these conditions are all due to yin vacuity and blood heat leading to mutual fanning of wind and fire. This then results in fire drafting phlegm upward. Since this medicinal is able to cool and generate blood, it subdues these evils.

Shi Wei (Folium Polypodii Linguae) is bitter and balanced. It mainly treats taxation heat evil qi and the five dribbling blocks.[194] It disinhibits urination by [dredging] the water passageways. Its other name is *Shi Zhe* (Stone Skin). It grows over rocks in the mountains and valleys.

Bai He (Bulbus Lilii)[195] is sweet and balanced. It mainly treats evil qi, abdominal distention, and heart pain. It disinihibits urination and defecation, supplements the center, and boosts the qi. It grows in rivers and valleys.

Zi Shen (Radix Salviae Chinensis)[196] is bitter and cold. It mainly treats accumulations and gatherings in the heart and abdomen and cold and heat evil qi. It frees the nine orifices and disinhibits urination and defecation. Its other name is *Mu Meng* (Female Usnea). It grows in mountains and valleys.

Wang Gua (Radix Trichosanthis Cucumeroidis)[197] is bitter and cold. It mainly treats wasting thirst, internal impediment, blood stasis, menstrual block, cold and heat, and aching pain. It boosts the qi and cures deafness. Its other name is *Tu Gua* (Earth Melon). It grows in plains and swamps.

---

[194] Urinary block is due to collection or stoppage of fluids. Since there are five kinds of fluid—sweat, urine, saliva, tears, and steam from the breath—there are five kinds of urinary block.

[195] Lily is able to move both the constructive and defensive and bring harmony between yin and yang. Nowadays, it is often used as a supplementing food.

[196] This medicinal is no longer used. Therefore, it is difficult to identify. Among the possibilities are Radix Polygoni Tenuicaulis and Radix Salviae Miltiorrhizae.

[197] This medicinal is often used to drain heat, move the blood, and expel stasis. In addition, it is able to precipitate water and promote lactation. Its indications include jaundice, wasting thirst, menstrual block, suppuration, swelling, lower abdominal fullness and pain, and urinary and fecal stoppage.

Da Huang (**Radix Et Rhizoma Rhei**)[198] is bitter, cold, and toxic. It mainly precipitates blood stasis, blood block, and cold and heat. It breaks concretions and conglomerations, accumulations and gatherings, and lodged rheum and abiding food. It flushes the stomach and intestines to weed out the stale and bring forth the new, disinhibits and frees the flow of water and grain, regulates the center to transform food, and quiets and harmonizes the five viscera. It grows in mountains and valleys.

Gan Sui (**Radix Euphorbiae Kansui**) is bitter, cold, and toxic. It mainly treats enlarged abdomen, mounting conglomeration, abdominal fullness, puffy swelling of the face and eyes, and lodged rheum and abiding food. It breaks concretions and hardness, accumulations and gatherings and disinhibits the water and grain passageways. Its other name is *Zhu Tian* (Governing Land). It grows in rivers and valleys.

Ting Li (**Semen Lepidii Seu Descurainiae**)[199] is acrid and cold. It mainly treats concretions, conglomerations, gatherings, and accumulation bound qi and [abiding] food and drink with cold and heat. It breaks hardness, expels evils, and disinhibits and frees the flow of the water passageways. Its other name is *Da Shi* (Great Room). Another name is *Da Shi* (Great Comfort). It grows in plains, swamps, and fields.

---

[198] Rhubarb is particularly able to drain damp heat and precipitate stagnation and accumulation. It is often used to treat cold damage, delirious speech with fever, malaria, dysentery, urinary and fecal stoppage, glomus pain, accumulations and gatherings, and jaundice. It is an indispensible medicinal for fire depressed in the blood and dryness of the stomach and intestines. In addition, it also treats phlegm, suppuration, swelling, ejection of blood, and nosebleed.

[199] There are two kinds of Lepidium, the sweet and bitter. Here, the author appears to only be referring to the bitter. Lepidium is especially good at downbearing the lung qi. Because the lung qi is the upper source of water, when it fails to descend, damp water flooding may occur giving rise to swelling, distention, phlegm cough, panting and chest fullness, etc. This is when this medicinal should be used.

Yuan Hua (**Flos Daphnis Genkwae**)[200]is bitter and warm. It is toxic, treating mainly cough and counterflow qi ascent, rales in the throat, panting, swollen throat, shortness of breath, *gu* toxins, ghosts, malaria, mounting conglomeration, welling abscesses, and swellings. It kills worms and fish. Its other name is *Qu Shui* (Water Eliminator). It grows in rivers and valleys.

Ze Qi (**Herba Euphorbiae Helioscopiae**)[201] is bitter and slightly cold. It mainly treats skin fever, enlarged abdomen due to water qi, puffy swelling of the limbs, face, and eyes, and, in males, yin qi insufficiency. It grows in rivers and swamps.

---

[200] This medicinal is woody rather than herbaceous. It is able to drastically precipitate water and, therefore, is often prescribed to treat various kinds of rheum and water problems. Its indications include the five rheums—lodged rheum, propping rheum, suspended rheum, hidden rheum, and spillage rheum. These rheum patterns may present various symptoms, such as panting and coughing, cold in the back, intestinal rumbling, diarrhea, propping fullness of the rib-side, and foaming at the mouth. The water patterns it is able to treat mainly include wind water, skin water, regular water, stone water, and yellow sweating. The common sign between these water troubles is edema, except for yellow sweating which is a type of jaundice.

[201] This is an important medicinal for abating fever, dispersing phlegm, and suppressing cough. It is able to disinhibit urination and defecation and thereby treat an enlarged abdomen. The word yin often refers to the genitals. Therefore, yin qi insufficiency here should be understood as impotence or lack of sexual desire.

70

Da Ji (Herba Seu Radix Cirsii Japonici)[202] is bitter and cold. It mainly treats *gu* toxins, the 12 waters,[203] abdominal fullness and acute pain, accumulations and gatherings, wind stroke, skin aching pain, and counterflow vomiting. Its other name is *Ang Ju* (Raised Hook).

Yao Hua (Flos Wikstroemiae Japonicae) is bitter and cold. It mainly treats cold damage and warm malaria, precipitates the 12 waters, breaks gatherings, accumulations, great hardness, concretions, and conglomerations, flushes abiding and aggregated food and drink away from the stomach and intestines as well as cold and heat evil qi, and disinhibits the water passageways. It grows in rivers and valleys.

Gou Wen (Herba Gelsemii Elegantis)[204] is acrid and warm. It mainly treats incised wounds, breast-feeding tetany, malign wind stroke,[205] cough and counterflow qi ascent, and water swelling. It kills demonic influx and *gu*

---

[202] This medicinal is able to drastically drain water. In addition, it is effective against phlegm rheum troubles. Li Shi-zhen (1518-1593 CE), the great pharmacologist, once explained this action of the medicinal in detail when he introduced the formula *Kong Xian Dan* (Drool-controlling Elixir). This is composed of *Da Ji* (Herba Seu Radix Cirsii Japonici), *Gan Sui* (Radix Euphorbiae Kansui), and *Bai Jie Zi* (Semen Sinapis Albae). He said:

> After phlegm drool has taken shape, entering the heart, it gives rise to withdrawal and epilepsy. Entering the lungs, it gives rise to cough, panting, and cold in the back. Entering the liver, it gives rise to rib-side pain, dry retching, and alternating cold and heat. Entering the channels and vessel networks, it gives rise to insensitivity and pain. Entering the sinews and bones, it gives rise to a contracting dull pain. Entering the skin and flesh, it gives rise to scrofulas, welling abscesses, and swellings... All these should be treated with *Kong Xian Dan* which will bring a miraculous effect.

[203] The 12 waters refer to all categories of swelling, for example, enlarged abdomen, swollen face, and swelling starting from below with a tendency to extend upward.

[204] *Gou Wen* (Herba Gelsemii Elegantis) is fatally poisonous. However, its true identity is controversial. Its Chinese name suggests that once any animal has a bite of it, it will die immediately.

[205] This implies hypertonicity of the limbs and tetany.

71

toxins. Its other name is *Ye Ge* (Wild Kudzu). It grows in the mountains and valleys.

Li Lu (**Radix Et Rhizoma Veratri**)[206] is acrid and cold. It is toxic, treating mainly *gu* toxins, cough and counterflow, diarrhea and dysentery, intestinal afflux, head sores, scabs, and malign sores. It kills various worms and eliminates dead muscles. Its other name is *Cong Ran* (Flourishing Scallion). It grows in mountains and valleys.

Wu Tou (**Radix Aconiti**)[207] is acrid and warm. It is toxic, treating mainly wind stroke and aversion to wind as after a soaking. It promotes sweating, eliminates cold damp impediment and cough and counterflow qi ascent, breaks accumulations and gatherings, and [relieves] cold and heat. The decoction of its juice is called *She Wang* (Shooting Net), and it can kill birds and beasts. Its other name is *Xi Du* (Extraordinary Toxin). Another name is *Ji Zi* (Immediate Child). It is also called *Wu Hui* (Black Beak). It grows in mountains and valleys.

---

[206] This medicinal is now used only as an emetic. If one is poisoned by it, Chinese Scallion can resolve it.

[207] *Wu Tou* (Radix Aconiti), *Tian Xiong* (Radix Lateralis Aconiti Carmichaeli), and *Fu Zi* (Radix Lateralis Praeparatus Aconiti Carmichaeli) are the same substance. In olden times, it was said that it was *Wu Tou* if collected in spring, *Fu Zi* if gathered in winter, and *Tian Xiong* if harvested in autumn. According to another definition, *Tian Xiong* is *Wu Tou* that is three inches or longer. Later, another distinction became popular. The main root was *Wu Tou*, while the lateral root was *Fu Zi* because the word *Fu* means attaching, lateral, etc.
The three medicinals have similar actions. The curative effects differ between *Wu Tou* and *Fu Zi* as follows. *Wu Tou* is particularly able to track down wind, overcome dampness, open obstinate phlegm, and cure intractable sores. In old prescriptions, *Wu Tou* was used more often than *Fu Zi*, especially when congestion and impediment (or qi and blood block) were concerned. Compared with it, *Fu Zi* is stronger in supplementing vacuity.

Tian Xiong (**Radix Lateralis Aconiti Carmichaeli**)[208] is acrid and warm. It mainly treats great wind, cold damp impediment, joint-running pain, hypertonicity, and slackness and tension. It breaks accumulations and gatherings, [treats] evil qi and incised wounds, fortifies the sinews and bones, and makes the body light and the walk strong. Its other name is *Bai Mu* (White Curtain). It grows in mountains and valleys.

Fu Zi (**Radix Lateralis Praeparatus Aconiti Carmichaeli**)[209] is acrid and warm. It is toxic. It mainly treats wind cold, cough and counterflow, and evil qi. It warms the center, [treats] incised wound, breaks concretions, hardness, accumulations, gatherings, and blood conglomerations, and [relieves] cold dampness, crippling wilt, hypertonicity, and pain in the knee with inability to walk. It grows in mountains and valleys.

Yang Zhi Zhu (**Flos Rhododendri Sinensis**) is acrid, warm, and toxic. It mainly treats bandit wind within the skin causing continual dull pain,

---

[208] See note 16 above. *Tian Xiong* is seldom used. It may help yang, warm the water viscera, *i.e.*, the kidneys, invigorate the lumbus and knees, boost the essence to brighten the eyes, free the orifices, and regulate the blood. It is good for wind and qi and, therefore, is used to treat wind cold damp impediment, water qi around the diaphragm in the chest, strings and aggregations (*i.e.*, masses in the abdomen), and sudden turmoil (*i.e.*, choleraic disease) with cramps, suppuration, and pain. It is also able to promote perspiration but also to stop sweating if it is massive.

[209] See note 16 above. This medicinal is able to reach all 12 channels and is able to vanquish all damp cold. Together with qi supplementing medicinals, it may restore original yang. Used in combination with blood supplementing medicinals, it is able to enrich and supplement kidney yin. It may also work together with effusing and dispersing medicinals to dispel wind cold from the exterior, while it is able to lead warm and hot medicinals to treat cold dampness in the interior. Therefore, it is often used to treat cold damage of the three yin, wind stroke, cough and counterflow, dysphagia-occlusion, qi and phlegm reversal cold of the limbs, spleen diarrhea, cold dysentery, sudden turmoil with cramps, hypertonicity, wind impediment, concretions and conglomerations, accumulations and gatherings, enduring fright epilepsy in children, welling and flat abscesses, and all hidden cold.
Fu Zi is used in two ways, uncooked and processed. The uncooked kind is strongly effusing; whereas the processed is particularly good at supplementing.

warm malaria, malign toxins, and various [kinds of] impediment. It grows in rivers and valleys.

Yin Yu (Folium Skimmiae Japonicae)[210] is bitter and warm. It mainly treats evil qi in the five viscera, cold and heat of the heart and abdomen with languor and emaciation, [cold and heat] which attack at regular intervals like malaria, and wind dampness impediment pain in various joints. It grows in rivers and valleys.

She Gan (Rhizoma Belamcandae Chinensis)[211] is bitter and balanced. It mainly treats cough and counterflow qi ascent, throat impediment, and sore throat affecting breathing. It disperses binding qi, counterflow evil in the abdomen, and great heat due to food and drink. Its other name is *Wu Shan* (Black Fan). Another name is *Wu Pu* (Black Palmtree Leaf). It grows in rivers and valleys.

Yuan Wei (Radix Iridis Tectori) is bitter and balanced. It mainly treats *gu* toxins and evil qi, demonic influx, and various toxins. It breaks concretions and conglomerations, accumulations and gatherings, removes water, and precipitates the three [kinds of] worms. It grows in mountains and valleys.

---

[210] Nowadays, this medicinal is seldom used. In olden times, it was prescribed as a ruling medicinal for treating wind epilepsy. This is either a kind of epilepsy with diverse signs or an epilepsy whose main manifestations are tremor of the extremities, head shaking, and clenched jaw.

[211] This medicinal is able to drain fire, disperse swelling, and resolve phlegm binding. It is often used to treat throat impediment, sore throat, chest fullness, abdominal distention, panting, menstrual block, constipation, mounting conglomeration, and mother of malaria. Mother of malaria is a kind of malaria complicated by inflammation of the spleen. In addition, it can be used to level the liver to brighten the eyes.

Guan Zhong (**Radix Aspidii Falcati**)[212] is bitter, slightly cold, and toxic. It mainly treats evil heat qi in the abdomen and various toxins. It kills the three [kinds of] worms. Its other name is *Guan Jie* (Running Through Joint). Another name is *Guan Qu* (Running Through Ditch). It is also called *Bai Tou* (Hundred Heads), *Hu Juan* (Tiger Roll), and *Bian Fu* (Flat Tally). It grows in mountains and valleys.

Fei Lian (**Flos Et Radix Carduntis Crispi**)[213] is bitter and balanced. It mainly treats heat in the bone joints and heaviness and aching pain in the lower legs. Protracted taking makes the body light. Its other name is *Fei Qing* (Lightly Flying). It grows in rivers and swamps.

Ban Xia (**Rhizoma Pinelliae Ternatae**)[214] is acrid and balanced. It mainly treats cold damage, cold and heat, and hardness below the heart. It downbears the qi, [treats] swollen and sore throat, head dizziness, chest distention, cough and counterflow, and rumbling intestines, and stops sweating. Its other name is *Di Wen* (Earth Texture). Another name is *Shui Yu* (Watery Jade). It grows in rivers and valleys.

---

[212] Several different plants supply this single-named medicinal depending on locale. Hsu identifies it as Rhizoma Blechni, while Bensky and Gamble identify it as any one of Rhizoma Dryopteridis Crassirhizomae, Rhizoma Woodawardiae Unigemmatae, Rhizoma Osmundiae Japonicae, or Rhizoma Matteucciae Struthiopteridis. It is believed that drinking water in which *Guan Zhong* has been dipped confers immunity during epidemics such as infectious hepatitis and measles. In addition, it cures head wind, flooding, vaginal discharge, postpartum abdominal pain and distention, and concretions and conglomerations.

[213] Nowadays, this medicinal is rarely if ever used, and its identity is problematic. Another likely plant is Crisium Ovalifolium. Because of the difficulty determining its identity, descriptions of its actions differ from scholar to scholar depending upon what actual species is used.

[214] This medicinal harmonizes the stomach and fortifies the spleen, supplements the liver and moistens the kidneys, moves water and eliminates dampness, opens depression and transforms phlegm, downbears the qi, disinhibits the water passageways, and restores the voice. Therefore, it is often prescribed to treat cold and heat in cold damage, dizziness, phlegm reversal, headache, supraorbital pain, sore throat, retching and vomiting, chest distention, abdominal fullness, goiters, and swelling.

Hu Zhang (**Rhizoma Arisaematis**) is bitter and warm. It is nontoxic, treating mainly heart pain, cold and heat, bound qi, accumulations and gatherings, lying beam,[215] injured sinews, [sinew] wilt, and contraction and slackening [of the sinews]. It disinhibits the water passageways. It grows in mountains and valleys.

Lang Dang Zi (**Semen Scopoliae Japonicae**)[216] is bitter and cold. It mainly treats toothache by driving out the worms, flesh impediment, and hypertonicity. It may make one walk briskly and behold ghosts. Taking [too] much of it may make one run frenetically. Protracted taking will make the body light, enabling one to run as fast as a galloping horse, fortify the will, boost the [physical] force, and enable one to communicate with spirits. Its other name is *Heng Tang* (Across the Road). It grows in rivers and valleys.

Shu Qi (**Herba Dichroae Febrifugae**) is acrid, balanced, and toxic. It mainly treats malaria, cough and counterflow, cold and heat, hard concretions and binding glomus in the abdomen, accumulation and gathering evil qi, *gu* toxins, and demonic influx. It grows in rivers and valleys.

---

[215] Lying beam is another name for heart accumulation and is one of the so-called five accumulations. It is mainly divided into two categories. One is a long mass below the heart accompanied by heart vexation. The other is a long mass starting from below the umbilicus which may extend up to below the heart.

[216] In olden times, the seed was used, but nowadays the root is prescribed instead. Scopolia Japonica is effective for strings and aggregations (*i.e.*, masses in the abdomen), cold qi in the abdomen, qi dysentery, prolapse of the rectum, and genital sweating. In addition, it is sometimes used to quiet the heart, settle the orientation, and expel wind. From the indications discussed in the text, this medicinal should be warm or hot rather than cold. The narration of its actions are also inconsistent. This suggests that this passage may have been garbled by unknown editors. For example, the statement that taking too much may make one run frenetically about is contradictory to the statement that protracted taking may make the body light. Medicinals which make the body light are typically classified as superior and, therefore, are without negative side effects.

76

Heng Shan (**Radix Dichroae Febrifugae**)[217] is bitter and cold. It mainly treats cold damage cold and heat, malaria due to heat, ghost toxins, bound phlegm in the chest, and counterflow vomiting. Its other name is *Hu Cao* (Dependent Weed). It grows in rivers and valleys.

Qing Xiang (**Herba Celosiae Argenteae**)[218] is bitter and slightly cold. It mainly treats evil qi, heat within the skin, and generalized wind itching. It kills the three [kinds of] worms. Its seed (Semen Celosiae Argenteae) is called *Cao Jue Ming* (Bright [Eye] Deciding Weed) and treats green-blue lips. Its other name is *Cao Hao* (Herbaceous Tall Stalk). Another name is *Lou Hao* (Crawling Tall Stalk). It grows in plains and valleys.

Lang Ya (**Radix Potentillae Cryptonis**) is bitter, cold, and toxic. It mainly treats evil qi, heat qi, scabs, malign sores, and hemorrhoids. It removes white worms [*i.e.*, pinworms]. Its other name is *Ya Zi* (Tooth). It grows in rivers and valleys.

Bai Lian (**Radix Ampelosis Serjaniaefaliae**)[219] is bitter and balanced. It mainly treats welling abscesses and flat abscesses, disperses bound qi, relieves pain, eliminates heat, and [treats] red eyes, fright epilepsy in

---

[217] The current name is *Chang Shan* which has the same implication as the old name *Heng Shan* in Chinese. *Heng Shan* gave way to *Chang Shan* simply because it violated an imperial name taboo. In feudal China, any name which sounded the same as the emperor's name had to be changed. Judging from the text, it seems that this medicinal is used to stop vomiting, but, as a matter of fact, it is more often prescribed to provoke vomiting. As an emetic, Radix Dichroae Febrifugae is able to expel the six kinds of phlegm—wind, cold, damp, heat, food, and qi phlegm—and clears the five categories of rheum—propping, lodged, suspended, spillage, and hidden rheum. In modern times, this medicinal is mostly used to treat malaria.

[218] Currently, this medicinal is used mainly for eye troubles which are not mentioned at all in the text. It is believed to be able to settle the liver and brighten the eyes as well as cure clear-eye blindness and red screen. It also treats bound heat following cold damage.

[219] This is an important medicinal for draining fire and dispersing binding. Nowadays, it is used mainly to treat various kinds of abscesses and sores, including clove sores, flat abscess effusion of the back, scalds and burns, incised wounds, scrofulas, sores, and hemorrhoids.

children, warm malaria, and, in females, genital swelling and pain. Its other name is *Tu He* (Cuscuta Kernel). Another name is *Bai Cao* (White Weed). It grows in mountains and valleys.

Bai Ji **(Rhizoma Bletillae Striatae)**[220] is bitter and balanced. It mainly treats welling abscesses and swellings, malign sores, putrid flat abscesses, damaged yin,[221] dead muscles, evil qi in the stomach, bandit wind, ghost stroke, and disablement of slackening and inability to contract. Its other name is *Gan Gen* (Sweet Root). Another name is *Lian Ji Cao* (Entangled Weed). It grows in rivers and valleys.

Cao Hao **(Herba Artemisiae Apiacae)**[222] is bitter and cold. It mainly treats scabies, itchy scabs, and malign sores, kills lice, [relieves] lodged heat in the joints, and brightens the eyes. Its other name is *Qing Hao* (Green Tall Stalk). Another name is *Fang Kui* (Opening). It grows in rivers and swamps.

Huan Jun **(Herba Phragmitis Communis)**[223] is salty and balanced. It mainly treats heart pain, warms the center, and removes long worms [*i.e.*, tapeworms], white crust, pinworms, snake and [insect] bite toxins, concretions and conglomerations, and various [other] worms. Its other name is *Huan Lu* (Damp Reed). It grows in pools and swamps.

---

[220] Currently, Bletilla has three uses. One is to treat damaged lungs causing lung bleeding. This typically manifests as coughing or hacking up of blood. Its second indication is bone fracture. Lastly, it is prescribed to treat burns, cracking of the skin, welling and flat abscesses, scrofulas, and hemorrhoids. However, in folk prescriptions, it is used to stop nosebleeding. For this purpose, it is applied externally, and it proves quite effective.

[221] Damaged yin means impotence in males and prolapse of the uterus in females.

[222] The current name is *Qing Hao*. In modern times, it is mainly used to clear heat to treat steaming bone taxation fever, postpartum vacuity fever, and warm malaria.

[223] Because this medicinal has been out of use for centuries, it is very hard to identify. It is possible that this is a species of mushroom growing in swamps or water margins.

Lian Qiao **(Fructus Forsythiae Suspensae)**[224] is bitter and balanced. It mainly treats cold and heat, mouse fistulas, scrofulas, welling abscesses and swellings, malign sores, goiters and tumors, bound heat, and *gu* toxins. Its other name is *Yi Qiao* (Strange Beauty). Another name is *Zhi* (Hub). It is also called *Jian Hua* (Orchid Flower), *She Gen* (Broken Root), and *San Lian* (Three Honesties). It grows in mountains and valleys.

Bai Tou Gong **(Radix Pulsatillae Chinensis)**[225] is bitter and warm. It is nontoxic, treating mainly warm malaria, mania, cold and heat, concretions and conglomerations, accumulations and gatherings, and goiter qi. It expels blood [stasis], relieves pain, and heals incised wound. Its other name is *Ye Zhang Ren* (Secluded Old Man). Yet another name is *Hu Wang Shi Zhe* (Envoy of the Nomad King). It grows in rivers and valleys.

Lu Ru **(Radix Euphorbiae Adenochlorae)** is sour and salty. It is toxic, treating mainly eroded and malign flesh, putrefying sores, and dead muscle. It kills scab worms, discharges pus and malign blood, and eliminates great wind, heat qi, forgetfulness, and melancholy. It grows in rivers and valleys.

---

[224] This medicinal is able to drain fire, eliminate damp heat, disperse congealed blood and gathered qi in various channels, disinhibit water, and free the flow of the channels. It is used to kill parasites, relieve pain, disperse swelling, discharge pus, and resolve toxins. In modern times, it is among the most frequently used medicinals for various sorts of sores.

[225] This medicinal is currently called *Bai Tou Weng*. Besides what is discussed in the text, Pulsatilla is able to treat all wind troubles, cold pain of the knees, nosebleed, baldness, and swollen testicles. In modern clinical practice, it is mainly used to treat dysentery.

Yang Tao (**Fructus Averrhoae Carambolae**)[226] is bitter and cold. It mainly treats fulminant fever, sudden generalized reddening, wind water,[227] accumulations and gatherings, and malign sores. It eliminates fever in children. Its other name is *Gui Tao* (Ghost Peach). Another name is *Yang Chang* (Goat Intestine). It grows in rivers and valleys.

Yang Ti (**Radix Rumicis Japonici**)[228] is bitter and cold. It mainly treats baldness and itchy scabs and eliminates fever and, in females, genital erosion. Its other name is *Dong Fang Xu* (East Constellation). Another name is *Lian Chong Lu* (Insect Linked Java Elder Fruit). It is also called *Gui Mu* (Ghost Eye). It grows in rivers and swamps.

Lu Huo (**Herba Rhynchosiae Volubilis**) is bitter and balanced. It mainly treats *gu* toxins, lumbar and abdominal pain and discomfort in females, intestinal abscesses, scrofulas, and sores. It grows in mountains and valleys.

Niu Bian (**Radix Aconiti Lycoctomi**) is bitter and slightly cold. It mainly treats skin sores and heat qi. It can be used to make bathwater. It kills gadflies and small worms. In addition, it treats cow diseases. It grows in rivers and valleys.

Lu Ying (**Flos Sambuci Japonici**) is bitter and cold. It mainly treats various impediments of the bones, hypertonicity and aching pain of the limbs, cold pain in the knees, impotence, shortness of breath, and swollen feet. It grows in rivers and valleys.

---

[226] Because this medicinal is never prescribed in modern times, its definite identity is not certain. Therefore, its Latin pharmacological identification should only be regarded as provisional. Other possibilities have been suggested.

[227] Wind water is generalized water swelling, which starts in the face and gradually extends to other parts with pain in the limb joints. This is usually complicated by fever and aversion to wind.

[228] Radix Rhei Undulati is an equally possible suggestion for the identity of this medicinal. It is usually used externally.

Jin Cao (**Herba Arthraxi Ciliaris**) is bitter and balanced. It mainly treats enduring cough and qi ascent, panting and counterflow, enduring cold, fright palpitations, scabs, bald white scalp sores, and sores. It kills small worms on the skin. It grows in rivers and valleys.

Xia Ku Cao (**Spica Prunellae Vulgaris**)[229] is bitter, acrid, and cold. It mainly treats cold and heat, scrofulas, mouse fistulas, and head sores. It breaks concretions, disperses goiter bound qi, [treats] swollen feet and damp impediment, and may make the body light. Its other name is *Xi Ju* (Slanting Bow). Another name is *Nai Dong* (Host). It grows in rivers and valleys.

Wu Jiu (**Herba Cotyledinis Malacophyllae**)[230] is sweet and cold. It mainly treats alternating skin cold and heat and disinhibits the small intestine and urinary bladder qi. It grows in mountains and valleys.

Zao Xiu (**Rhizoma Paridis Polyphyllae Seu Tetraphyllae**)[231] is bitter and slightly cold. It mainly treats fright epilepsy, shaking of the head and worrying tongue, heat qi in the abdomen, madness, welling abscesses, sores, and genital erosion. It precipitates the three [kinds of] worms and removes snake toxins. Its other name is *Zhe Xiu* (End of Stinging). It grows in rivers and valleys.

Shi Chang Sheng (**Herba Adianfi Monochlamydis**) is salty and slightly cold. It mainly treats cold and heat, malign sores, and great heat and

---

[229] This medicinal is able to resolve internal heat and mollify liver fire. It has proved to be quite effective for some eye disorders, especially distention of the eyes, high pressure in the eyes, tearing, aversion to light, and eye pain. In summer, it is often used to prevent and treat prickly heat.

[230] There is as yet no consensus concerning the identity of this medicinal. Therefore, this identification is only provisional.

[231] This medicinal boosts the spleen and upbears the clear qi of the stomach. It ascends to the lungs to boost the blood and move the qi, and it invigorates the kidneys to boost the essence. It quickens the blood, stops bleeding, disperses swelling, and resolves toxins.

wards off ghost qi and ill matters. Its other name is *Dan Cao* (Cinnabar Weed). It grows in mountains and valleys.

Lang Du (**Radix Galarhoei Eblactealati**) is acrid and balanced. It mainly treats cough and counterflow qi ascent, breaks drink and food accumulations and gatherings, and [relieves] cold and heat, water qi, malign sores, mouse fistulas, flat abscess, erosion [of flesh], ghosts, spirits, and *gu* toxins. It kills birds and beasts. Its other name is *Xu Du* (Succeeding Toxin). It grows in mountains and valleys.

Gui Jiu (**Radix Podophylli Versipellis**) is acrid and warm. It mainly kills *gu* toxins, demonic influx, and spiritual matters. It keeps off malign qi and ill matters, expels evils, and resolves hundreds of toxins. Its other name is *Jiao Xi* (Rhinoceros Horn). Another name is *Ma Mu Du Gong* (Horse Eye Toxic Master). It is also called *Jiu Jiu* (Nine Mortars). It grows in mountains and valleys.

Bian Xu (**Herba Polygoni Avicularis**)[232] is bitter and balanced. It mainly treats wet spreading sores, itchy scabs, flat abscesses, and hemorrhoids. It kills the three [kinds of] worms. It grows in mountains and valleys.

Shang Lu (**Radix Phytolaccae Acinosae**)[233] is acrid and balanced. It mainly treats water distention, mounting conglomeration, and impediment, irons out welling abscesses and swellings, and kills ghosts and spiritual matters. Its other name is *Chang Gen* (Withered Root). Another name is *Ye Hu* (Night Crying). It grows in rivers and valleys.

---

[232] Currently, this medicinal is often used to kill roundworms and treat strangury, malign (*i.e.*, intractable) sores, and jaundice.

[233] Phytolacca is a drastic water-precipitating medicinal able to eliminate damp heat and cure water swelling. Besides the indications discussed in the text, it is also used to cure throat impediment and induce abortion.

Nu Qing **(Herba Metaplexis Stauntoni)**[234] is acrid and balanced. It mainly treats *gu* toxins, expels evil and malign qi, kills ghosts and warm malaria, and keeps off ill matters. Its other name is *Que Piao* (Bird Gourd Ladle). It grows in mountains and valleys.

Bai Fu Zi **(Rhizoma Typhonii Gigantei)**[235] mainly treats heart pain, blood impediment, and hundreds of diseases in the face. It is able to carry the strength of [other] medicinals.[236] It grows in Shu Prefecture [or what is now Sichuan province].

Gu Huo **(Semen Abutilonis Seu Malvae)**[237] is sweet and warm. It mainly treats great wind, evil qi, damp impediment, and cold pain. Protracted taking may make the body light, increase life span, and slow aging. Its other name is *Dong Kui Zi* (Winter Big Flower Seed). It grows in rivers and swamps.

Bie Ji[238] is bitter and slightly warm. It mainly treats wind, cold, damp impediment, generalized heaviness, aching pain in the limbs, and cold evil joint-running pain. It grows in rivers and valleys.

---

[234] In olden times, the root (Radix Metaplexis Stauntoni) may have been used instead.

[235] Currently, this medicinal is often used as a face cream to remove patches, blemishes, papules, etc. It is also prescribed for genital itching.

[236] This implies that Typhonium is able to lead other medicinals upward. Depending on which other medicinals it is combined with, it treats a variety of troubles, such as paralysis, wind phlegm dizziness, hemilateral headache, phlegm inversal headache, lockjaw, throat impediment, and pain and swelling of the throat.

[237] This medicinal has long been out of clinical use.

[238] Because this medicinal has been out of use for centuries, it is now unidentifiable. It is only known to have been a weed growing in the mountains.

Shi Xia Chang Qing **(Herba Seu Radix Cynanchi Paniculati)**[239] is salty and balanced. It mainly treats demonic influx, spiritual matters, and evil and malign qi. It kills hundreds of spirits, *gu* toxins, and old demonic influx and transformation [manifesting as] running about, crying, sadness, and abstraction. Its other name is *Xu Chang Qing* (Senior Minister Xu). It grows in pools and swamps.

Qiao Gen **(Radix Forsythiae Suspensae)**[240] is bitter and cold. It mainly precipitates heat qi, boosts yin essence, makes the facial complexion attractive, and brightens the eyes. Protracted taking may make the body light and slow aging. It grows in plains and swamps.

Qu Cao[241] is bitter. It mainly treats chest and rib-side pain, evil qi, cold and heat in the intestines, and yin impediment.[242] Protracted taking may make the body light, boost the qi, and slow aging. It grows in rivers and swamps.

---

[239] This medicinal is currently called *Xu Chang Qing*.

[240] Because this medicinal fell out of use by at least the 7th century CE, its identity is now uncertain. The pharmacological identification given here should only be regarded as provisional.

[241] The translator has failed to identify this medicinal.

[242] Yin impediment means painful impediment. In this case, pain in the joints is its most outstanding characteristic. According to another interpretation, this refers to impediment primarily caused by cold.

Woods: Superior Class

Fu Ling **(Sclerotium Poriae Cocos)**[243] is sweet and balanced. It mainly

---

[243] Poria quiets the heart and spirit, boosts the qi, regulates the constructive and defensive, boosts the spleen, drains the lungs, and drains damp heat from the bladder. In his exposition on this passage, Xu Da-chun (1693-1771 CE) ascribed all the troubles of chest and rib-side counterflow qi, worry and indignation, binding and pain below the heart, cold and heat, cough and counterflow, etc. to the spleen being too vacuous to transform water. Then he said:

> To treat rheum, bland [flavored medicinals] may effect disinhibition. On the contrary, if a heavy medicinal is prescribed, it may be repelled, unable to penetrate. Poria is very light and bland. It is ascribed to earth, and earth overcomes water. Therefore, it is able to dredge and flush [water] away through urination.

On this point, Chen Xiu-yuan agreed. He said:

> Poria enters the lungs and spleen. The chest is the seat of the lungs, and the rib-side is the region where the spleen is located. When the qi there counterflows upward, it gives rise to worry, indignation, evil fright, and fearful palpitations. The seven affects are out of harmony. If water evils collect in the region below the heart, they will give rise to binding pain. If water qi is not transformed, vexatious fullness will arise. If this overwhelms the *tai yin*, cough and counterflow will arise. If this is held up in the constructive and defensive, fever and aversion to cold will arise. If rheum is retained internally, fluids and humors will not ascend. Then this will lead to parched mouth and dry tongue. All these illnesses cannot be healed unless urination is harmonized [*i.e.*, disinhibited] to make water move so that the qi is enabled to transform [water].

There are two kinds of Poria, white and red. *Bai Fu Ling* (Sclerotium Album Poriae Cocos) tends to supplement, while *Chi Fu Ling* (Sclerotium Rubrum Poriae Cocos) is stronger for draining damp heat. In the premodern literature, if the type of Poria
(continued...)

treats chest and rib-side counterflow qi, binding and pain below the heart due to worry, indignation, fright, and fear,[244] cold and heat, vexatious fullness, cough and counterflow, and parched mouth and dry tongue. It disinhibits urination. Protracted taking may quiet the ethereal soul, nourish the spirit, make one free from hunger, and prolong life. Its other name is *Fu Tu* (Crouching Rabbit). It grows in mountains and valleys.

Song Zhi (**Resina Pini**)[245] is bitter and warm. It mainly treats welling and flat abscesses, malign sores, head sores, bald white scalp sores, itchy scabs, and wind qi. It quiets the five viscera and eliminates heat. Protracted taking may make the body light and prolong life. Its other name is *Song Gao* (Pine Paste). Yet another name is *Song Zhi* (Pine Tallow). It grows in mountains and valleys.

Bai Shi (**Semen Biotae Orientalis**)[246] is sweet and balanced. It mainly

---

[243](...continued)
was not mentioned, then the white variety was meant. In addition, *Fu Shen* (Sclerotium Pararadicis Poriae Cocos) is also implied in this discussion. It is specifically effective for quieting the spirit and stabilizing the heart. *Fu Ling Pi* (Cortex Sclerotii Poriae Cocos) is also commonly used. It is particularly good at moving water to treat water swelling.

[244] The phrase from binding to fear may be rendered in another way. Then we may have, "binding and pain below the heart, and worry, indignation, etc." See note 1 above to understand the implications of this change in reading.

[245] In modern clinical practice, Pine Resin is only used externally and is seldom prescribed for oral administration.

[246] The current name of this medicinal is *Bai Zi Ren* or *Bai Ren*. In an annotation on this passage, Ye Gui said:

Biota Seeds enter the heart and treat fright palpitations. Their qi is balanced. Therefore, they boost the lung qi. Their flavor is sweet. So they [also] boost the spleen qi. They are able to enrich, moisten, and boost the heart qi. To treat wind, one should first treat the blood. Once the blood is moved, wind will die out on its own. Biota Seeds boost spleen blood. Once the blood is moved and wind has died down, the spleen will become strong and comfortable. It follows that dampness is precipitated. Biota Seeds are
(continued...)

treats fright palpitations, quiets the five viscera, boosts the qi, and eliminates wind damp impediment. Protracted taking may render the facial complexion shiny and attractive, sharpen the ears and eyes, and make one free from hunger, never senile, and the body light while prolonging life. It grows in mountains and valleys.

Jun Gui (**Cortex Cinnamomi Cassiae**)[247] is acrid and warm. It mainly treats

---

[246](...continued)
balanced [of qi] and sweet. Thus they boost yin. When yin is made abundant, the five viscera will become quiet... Nowadays, they are used as a medicinal to please the spleen, nourish the heart, moisten the kidneys, enrich the liver, sharpen the wits, and quiet the spirit.

[247] In olden times, there was a certain amount of confusion surrounding the distinction between *Jun Gui* and *Mu Gui* (next passage). Li Shi-zhen considered these different plants. However, according to Chen Cang-qi, a pharmacologist of the Tang dynasty, they are the same plant but, in terms of their use as medicinals, are different in quality. Practically speaking, they are the same substance, *i.e.*, the bark of cinnamon. The thick bark is *Mu Gui*, while the thin bark is *Jun Gui*. In modern prescriptions, there is a distinction between *Rou Gui* (also called *Guan Gui*), *Gui Zhi*, and *Gui Xin*. *Rou Gui* is the Cinnamon Bark which is thick and purplish. *Gui Zhi* is the bark of the tender Cinnamon Twig, while *Gui Xin* is shaved Cinnamon Bark.

Rou Gui (a.k.a. *Guan Gui*) is acrid and sweet and very hot of qi. It supplements the lower burner and life gate ministerial fire and boosts the kidneys. It suppresses cough and counterflow qi ascent, promotes perspiration, dredges the blood vessels, and removes wind cold from the constructive and defensive. In addition, it treats abdominal cold pain, diarrhea due to overwhelming dampness, choleraic disease with cramps, yang vacuity spontaneous sweating, headache, red eyes, and dead fetus. It is often used as a conductor for various medicinals.

Gui Zhi is acrid and sweet in flavor and warm of qi. It warms the channels and frees the flow of the vessels, promotes perspiration and resolves the muscles, disinhibits the lung qi, and dissipates blood amassment in the lower burner. It treats cold damage headache, wind stroke spontaneous sweating, painful wind (*i.e.*, rheumatic arthritis), and rib-side wind pain.

Gui Xin is bitter and acrid. It is able to lead the blood to transform pus and turn the blood into sweat. As such, it is an important medicinal to draw the toxins of
(continued...)

hundreds of diseases, nurtures the essence spirit, and renders the facial complexion harmonious. It may serve as an usher or envoy for various medicinals. Protracted taking may make the body light, prevent senility, and render the face bright and efflorescent, thus forever looking charming like a child's face. It grows in the mountains and valleys of Jiao Zhi.[248]

Mu Gui (Cortex Cinnamomi Cassiae)[247] is acrid and warm. It mainly treats cough and counterflow qi ascent, binding qi, throat impediment, and [inhibited] breathing. It disinhibits the joints, supplements the center, and boosts the qi. Protracted taking may enable one to communicate with spirits, make the body light, and prevent senility. It grows in mountains and valleys.

Du Zhong (Cortex Eucommiae Ulmoidis)[249] is acrid and balanced. It

---

[247](...continued)
welling and flat abscesses and pox sores from the inside. Moreover, it disperses stasis, promotes the growth of the muscles (*i.e.*, flesh), supplements taxation, joins severed sinews, and warms the lumbus and knees. It treats all kinds of heart pain, wind impediment, concretions and conglomerations, dysphagia-occlusion, and abdominal pain. In many cases, *Rou Gui* is used as a substitute for it.

[248] *I.e.*, present-day Guangxi Province

[249] Eucommia is sweet and slightly acrid in flavor and warm of qi. Sweetness and acridity are able to supplement, while slight acridity moistens. Therefore, this medicinal supplements and moistens liver yin, and hence Eucommia is the right choice for lumbago and knee pain due to kidney vacuity, not to wind cold. Wang Ang (1615-? CE) said:

Because the child is able to make the mother replete, Eucommia supplements the kidneys at the same time [as the liver]. When the liver is replenished, the sinews will become strong, and, when the kidneys are replenished, the bones will become hard. [Therefore, this medicinal] is able to produce affinity between the sinews and bones.

However, concerning the actions of Eucommia, Ye Gui took a different approach. He said:

Eucommia boosts the lungs. Lung metal generates kidney water. For that
(continued...)

mainly treats pain in the lumbus and knees, supplements the center, boosts the essence qi, fortifies the sinews and bones, strengthens the will, and eliminates genital damp itch and dribbling after voiding. Protracted taking may make the body light and slow aging. Its other name is *Si Xian* (Missing the Immortal). It grows in mountains and valleys.

Man Jing Shi (**Fructus Viticis**)[250] is bitter and slightly cold. It mainly treats cold and heat in the sinews and bones, damp impediment, and hypertonicity. It brightens the eyes, fortifies the teeth, disinhibits the nine orifices, and eliminates white worms [*i.e.*, pinworms]. Protracted taking may make the body light and slow aging. This is true of *Xiao Jing Shi* (Semen Viticis Negundi).[251]

---

[249](...continued)
reason, it relieves pain in the lumbus and knees. The lungs are the source of fluids. Because it can make yin adundant, it supplements the center. The lungs govern the qi and generate water. This is why it boosts the essence and qi. Once the essence and qi are boosted, the liver will have no lack of blood to nourish the sinews and the kidneys will have no lack of marrow to fill the bones. As a result, it fortifies the sinews and the bones. The lungs govern the qi. When the lungs are boosted, the qi becomes unyielding and prodigious. In consequence, the will becomes strong. [Genital] damp itching is due to dampness. Since Eucommia moistens the lungs, it may free the water passageways. Then dampness is moved. It boosts the lung qi. Once the qi is made secure, it is able to contain the essence so that dribbling after voiding is cured.

[250] The current name of this medicinal is *Man Jing Zi*. It cools the blood, tracks wind, and eliminates dampness. It treats damp impediment and hypertonicity since these troubles are caused by accumulation of cold, heat, and dampness. Eye and tooth disorders are usually due to heat, wind, and dampness. Therefore, they are also indications of this medicinal.

[251] In modern prescriptions, Succus or Lignum Viticis Negundi are usually used instead of Semen Viticis Negundi. For killing parasites, Vitex Trifolia is not as frequently used as Vitex Negundum. At the end of this passage, some versions have a sentence, "It grows in mountains and valleys."

Nu Zhen Shi (Fructus Ligustri Lucidi)[252] is bitter and balanced. It mainly supplements the center, quiets the five viscera, and nurtures the essence spirit. It is able to eliminate hundreds of diseases. Protracted taking may make one fat and strong and the body light and prevent senility. It grows in rivers and valleys.

Sang Shang Ji Sheng (Ramulus Loranthi Seu Visci)[253] is bitter and balanced. It mainly treats lumbago, rigidity of the back in children, and welling abscesses and swellings. It quiets the fetus, replenishes the muscles and skin, fortifies the teeth and hair, and promotes the growth of the beard and eyebrows. Its seed [Semen Loranthi Seu Visci] brightens the eyes, makes the body light, and enables one to communicate with spirits. Its other name is *Ji Xue* (Parasitic Dust). Yet another name is *Yu Mu* (Abiding Wood). It is also called *Wan Tong* (Naughty Child). It grows in mountains and valleys.

Su He (Semen Prinsepiae Uniflorae)[254] is sweet and balanced. It is nontoxic, mainly treating heart and abdominal evil binding qi and brightening the eyes. [It also treats] red, painful, wounded eyes, and tearing. Protracted taking may make the body light, boost the qi, and make one free from hunger. It grows in rivers and valleys.

---

[252] The current name of this medicinal is *Nu Zhen Zi*.

[253] The current name of this medicinal is *Sang Ji Sheng*. It is mainly used for strengthening the kidneys and boosting the blood. Once the kidneys are made strong, the lumbus will become strong and the teeth secure. Once the blood is boosted, the fetus will naturally become quiet.

[254] The current name of this medicinal is *Su Ren*. Prinsepia Seeds nourish the blood, disperse wind, and dissipate heat. In modern prescriptions, they are mainly used for various eye diseases. In addition, they treat bound phlegm glomus and deep-source nasal congestion.

Bai Mu **(Cortex Phellodendri)**[255] is bitter and cold. It mainly treats binding qi and heat in the five viscera and the intestines and stomach, jaundice, and intestinal hemorrhoids. It treats diarrhea and dysentery, leaking and red and white [vaginal discharge] in females, and genital erosion sores in males and females. Its root [Radix Phellodendri] is called *Tan Huan* (Sandalwood Pillar). It grows in mountains and valleys.

Xin Yi **(Flos Magnoliae Liliflorae)**[256] is acrid and warm. It mainly treats cold and heat of the five viscera and generalized [cold and heat], head wind, pain in the brain, and black patches on the face. Protracted taking may precipitate the qi, make the body light and the eyes bright, increase longevity, and slow aging. Its other name is *Xin Yin* (Acrid Conductor). Yet another name is *Hou Tao* (Throat Peach). It is also called *Fang Mu* (House Wood). It grows in rivers and valleys.

Yu Pi **(Cortex Ulmi Pumilae)**[257] is sweet and balanced. It mainly treats urinary and fecal stoppage, disinhibits the water passageway, and eliminates evil qi. Protracted taking may make the body light and the person free from hunger. Its fruit [Fructus Ulmi Pumilae] is even better [for the above troubles]. Its other name is *Ling Yu* (Withering Elm Tree). It grows in mountains and valleys.

---

[255] The current name of this medicinal is *Huang Bai*. Phellodendron is acrid and bitter. Bitterness fortifies the kidneys, while acridity moistens them. In addition, it drains bladder fire. It is also an important medicinal for clearing damp heat from the five viscera and the stomach and intestines as well. The indications explained in the text are all illnesses due to damp heat. Moreover, it is able to treat wilting and jaundice.

[256] This medicinal helps the clear yang of the stomach ascend to reach the head. Therefore, it treats head wind, various nasal disorders, etc. In addition, it warms the center, resolves the muscles, disinhibits the joints, and frees the flow of the blood vessels.

[257] Elm Bark is a disinihibitor, able to move the channels and vessels. It treats dead fetus in the womb, the five kinds of strangury, and various sores. However, in modern clinical practice, it is mainly prescribed to treat insomnia.

Suan Zao (Semen Zizyphi Spinosae)[258] is sour and balanced. It mainly treats heart and abdominal cold and heat and evil binding qi, aching pain in the limbs, and damp impediment. Protracted taking may quiet the five viscera, make the body light, and prolong life. It grows in rivers and swamps.

Huai Zi (Semen Sophorae Japonicae)[259] is bitter and cold. It mainly treats evil qi and heat in the five internals,[260] stops drooling and spitting, supplements expiry and damage, and [cures] the five kinds of hemorrhoids, burns, and, in females, mammary conglomeration and acute pain of the child's viscus [*i.e.*, the uterus]. It grows in plains and swamps.

---

[258] Zizyphus Spinosa is a very important medicinal for treating insomnia because it supplements the liver and gallbladder and is also able to fortify the spleen. When the liver is vacuous, the gallbladder must also be vacuous. All the viscera and bowels count on the gallbladder for decision-making. If the gallbladder suffers insufficiency, the heart is restless, and, when there is liver vacuity, it is hard for the corporeal soul to find a place in which to reside. As a result, sleeplessness arises.

[259] Nowadays, the flower and the pod (Flos Immaturus or Fructus Sophorae Japonicae) are commonly used, and the seed is rarely used as a medicinal. Sophora Flower moistens liver dryness, clears lung fire, and cools the large intestine. Once metal is debilitated, it is surely subjected to the bullying of fire. If the lungs and large intestine are attacked by fire, Sophora Flower or Fruit may clear this, thus putting the lungs and large intestine at rest. Therefore, this is an important medicinal for hemorrhoids, intestinal wind, etc.

[260] In this phrase, the five internals refer to the five viscera. Evils in the lungs give rise to drooling and copious sputum, while those in the liver lead to expiry and damage of the vessel network. Fire sores are ascribed to evil qi in the heart. Evil qi of the spleen is the cause of mammary conglomeration. Abdominal hypertonicity and pain is impugned to evil qi in the kidneys. Because Sophora Flower or Fruit is able to clear evil heat qi from the five viscera, all these illnesses may be cured.

Gou Qi (**Lycium Chinensis**)[261] is bitter and cold. It mainly treats evil qi in the five internals, center heat, wasting thirst, and generalized impediment. Protracted taking may fortify the sinews and bones, make the body light, and slow aging. Its other name is *Qi Gen* (Root of Lycium). Yet another name is *Di Gu* (Earth Bone). It is also called *Gou Ji* (Temporary Abstention) and *Di Fu* (Earth Assistant). It grows in plains and swamps.

Ju You (**Citrus**)[262] is acrid and warm. It mainly treats concretions and heat

---

[261] The word *Gou Qi* here refers to the fruit, the stem, and/or the root bark of Lycium Chinensis. One should note that Lycium Berries are not bitter but sweet. Generally speaking, this passage is mainly concerned with *Di Gu Pi* (Cortex Radicis Lycii Chinensis) as it is currently called. *Di Gu Pi* downbears lung fire, drains liver and kidney vacuity heat, cools the blood, and supplements the righteous qi. In clinical practice, it is often used to abate heat or fever, particularly steaming bones. The fruit (*Gou Qi Zi*, Fructus Lycii Chinensis) enriches the kidneys, moistens the lungs, clears the liver, and supplements the heart. It is a medicinal for generating the essence and invigorating yang. It fortifies the sinews and bones and brightens the eyes.

[262] The words *Ju You* do not merely refer to Citrus Reticulatae but the whole category of Citrus, including Citrus Nobilis, Citrus Medicae, etc. In modern times, only the peel and seeds are commonly used as medicinals.

Ju Pi, also called *Chen Pi* (Pericarpium Citri Reticulatae), regulates the center, frees the diaphragm, abducts stagnation, disperses phlegm, disinhibits water, and disperses binding. All these actions are attributed to its nature of drying dampness and precipitation of the qi. Chen Xiu-yuan said:

> Because it enters the lungs, it mainly treats conglomerations and counterflow qi above the diaphragm. Because it enters the liver, it disinhibits water and grain. Because it enters the heart, it makes the sovereign fire bright and removes the foul qi of the turbid yin.

The reason for these effects is this medicinal's precipitation of the qi. In modern prescriptions, it is often used to fortify the spleen and open the stomach, normalize the qi and disperse food, eliminate phlegm and resolve chest impediment. In addition, it is able to cure diarrhea and dysentery. *Ju Hong* (Exocarpium Citri Erythrocarpae) is most often used to precipitate the qi and disperse phlegm. *Qing Pi* (Pericarpium Citri Reticulatae Viride) has similar actions as *Chen Pi*. It is mainly used to break concretions and conglomerations, glomus, and bound heat. *Ju He*

(continued...)

counterflow qi in the chest. It also disinhibits water and grain. Protracted taking may remove foul breath, precipitate the qi, and enable one to communicate with spirits. Its other name is *Ju Pi* (Pericarpium Citri Reticulatae). It grows in the mountains, rivers, and valleys of the South.

---

[262](...continued)
(Semen Citri) transforms phlegm and dissipates binding (*i.e.*, scatters nodulation) and treats mounting pain.

Woods: Middle Class

Gan Qi (**Lacca Sinica Exsiccata**)[263] is acrid and warm. It is nontoxic, mainly treating expiry and damage. It supplements the center, joins [broken] sinews and bones, fills the marrow and brain, quiets the five viscera, and [treats] five slows and six fasts[264] as well as wind cold damp impediment. *Sheng Qi* (liquid Lacquer) removes long worms [*i.e.*, tapeworms]. Protracted taking may make the body light and slow aging. It grows in rivers and valleys.

Mu Lan (**Cortex Magnoliae Obovatae**) is bitter and cold.[265] It mainly treats great generalized fever within the skin, removes heat red boils in the face

---

[263] Lacquer is toxic. It moves the blood, kills worms, and disperses accumulations and gatherings. It is no longer used in modern prescriptions.

[264] The five slows probably refer to retarded growth in children, *i.e.*, slowness in acquiring the ability to stand, walk, and speak and slowness in growing teeth and head hair. The word *ji* (fast, hasty) may also mean extreme. In that case, the six extremes mean extreme debility of the sinews, bones, blood, flesh, essence, and qi. However, we have translated this term here as the six fasts in order to maintain the yin-yang logic of the original Chinese words, juxtaposing the five slows with the six fasts.

[265] In modern clinical practice, this medicinal is mainly prescribed for various dermatoses.

and drinker's nose, and [heals] malign wind, *lai* disease,[266] and genital damp itch. It [also] brightens the eyes. Its other name is *Lin Lan* (Forest Orchid). It grows in mountains and valleys.

Long Yan (Arillus Euphoriae Longanae)[267] is sweet and balanced. It mainly treats evil qi in the five viscera, quiets the will, and [relieves] aversion to food. Protracted taking may strengthen the ethereal soul, sharpen [the ears and eyes], make the body light, prevent senility, and enable one to communicate with the spirit light. Its other name is *Yi Zhi* (Wits Sharpener). It grows in mountains and valleys.

Hou Po (Cortex Magnoliae Officinalis)[268] is bitter and warm. It is

---

[266] *Lai* is the traditional Chinese name for leprosy and is characterized by insensitivity of the limbs, fever in the limb joints, weakness of the hands and feet, hoarse voice, blurred vision, and pricking pain in the focus. There are two species of *lai*, the white and the red. In the white species, there is whitening of the skin, while in the red, there is erythema.

[267] The current name of this medicinal is *Gui Yuan*. It is sweet in flavor and warm of qi. It nourishes the heart, supplements the blood, opens the stomach, and boosts the spleen. It is often prescribed to treat thought and worry taxation damage, forgetfulness, fearful throbbing, and intestinal wind with hemafecia. In olden times, Longans were often confused with *Yi Zhi* (Fructus Alpiniae Oxyphyllae) which is acrid. This medicinal is included in the wood section instead of the fruit section because, in ancient times, it was thought to be inedible.

[268] Magnolia Bark is able to eliminate dampness and flush away repletion with a sweeping force. Therefore, it is an important medicinal for relieving chest and abdominal fullness and distention. In addition, it is often used to level the stomach and regulate the center, disperse phlegm and transform food, move bound water and break dead blood, kill worms and check stomach reflux, relieve abdominal cold pain and cure diarrhea and dysentery, suppress cough and panting, and overcome choleraic disease.

Magnolia Bark is not a specific medicinal for exterior pathoconditions, but it is inclined to work towards the exterior. Therefore, in this passage, it is said to cure conditions such as wind stroke, cold damage, and headache. Moreover, in combination with different medicinals, it may bring different effects. Wang Hao-gu said:

(continued...)

nontoxic, mainly treating wind stroke, cold damage, headache, cold and heat, fright qi, blood impediment, and dead muscles. It removes the three [kinds of] worms. It grows in mountains and valleys.

***Zhu Ye* (Folium Bambusae)**[269] is bitter and balanced. It mainly treats cough and counterflow qi ascent, spillage sinew hypertonicity,[270] and malign sores. It kills small worms. Its root [Radix Bambusae], when decocted, can boost the qi, quench thirst, supplement vacuity, and precipitate the qi. Its sap [Succus Bambusae] mainly treats wind tetany and wind impediment. Its seed [Semen Bambusae] may enable one to communicate with the spirit light, make the body light, and boost the qi.

---

[268](...continued)
Used together with Immature Citrus Aurantium and Rhubarb, it drains repletion fullness. Used together with Orange Peel and Atractylodes, it eliminates dampness fullness. Used together with resolving disinhibitors, it treats cold damage and headache. Used together with draining disinhibitors, it thickens [*i.e.*, fortifies] the stomach and intestines. Roughly speaking, it is bitter in flavor and warm in nature. Bitterness can be used to drain, while warming can be used to supplement.

[269] Because there is more than one species of bamboo, this medicinal may also be described as sweet and cool. However, these species, though different, have similar actions. Bamboo Leaves cool the heart, moderate the spleen, and eliminate wind evils in the upper burner. These actions account for their indications such as vexatious heat, thirst, fever, congesting heat phlegm, cough and panting, ejection of blood, sudden loss of voice, fright epilepsy in children, and retching and vomiting. Bamboo Sap is extracted through heating a freshly cut piece of bamboo over a small fire. It is able to treat clenched jaw, wind tetany, withdrawal and mania, vexation and restlessness, stirred fetus, etc. Bamboo Root and Bamboo Seed are now seldom used.

[270] The meaning of the word spillage in the expression, "spillage sinew hypertonicity," is opaque. The translator has failed to make out its meaning. Some scholars suspect it as a typographical error for cure.

Zhi Shi (Fructus Immaturus Citri Aurantii)[271] is bitter and cold. It mainly treats great wind within the skin giving rise to tormenting itching as if [caused by] flax seeds, eliminates cold and heat and heat binding, stops dysentery, promotes the growth of the muscles and flesh, disinhibits the five viscera, boosts the qi, and makes the body light. It grows in river and swamps.

Shan Zhu Yu (Fructus Corni Officinalis)[272] is sour. It is nontoxic, mainly treating evil qi below the heart and cold and heat. It warms the center, expels cold damp impediment, and removes the three [kinds of] worms. Protracted taking may make the body light. Its other name is *Shu Zao* (Shu Date). It grows in mountains and valleys.

Wu Zhu Yu (Fructus Evodiae Rutecarpae)[273] is acrid and warm. It mainly

---

[271] Actually, this passage covers two medicinals—*Zhi Shi* (Fructus Immaturus Citri Aurantii) and *Zhi Ke* (Fructus Citri Aurantii). In olden times, there was a sophisticated discrimination between these two in terms of their actions. In fact, they have similar curative effects. The only difference is that the action of the unripe fruit is more drastic than that of the ripe fruit. Bitter Orange breaks the qi. Once the qi is moved, the blood will enjoy free circulation. In consequence, phlegm will be dispersed, panting suppressed, glomus and distention eliminated, pricking pain relieved, and pressure in the rectum resolved. On that account, it is an important medicinal in the treatment of chest impediment, chest binding, phlegm aggregation, concretions and conglomerations, counterflow retching, cough, rib-side distention, diarrhea, dysentery, intestinal wind, and hemorrhoids. Besides, it is also able to open the stomach and disperse food accumulation.

[272] Cornus warms and supplements the liver and kidneys and fortifies yin and secures yang. Therefore, it warms the lumbus and knees, constrains urination, and promotes sweating. In addition to the indications explained in the text, it treats wind cold impediment, nasal congestion, yellowing of the eyes, ringing in the ears, deafness, and boils on the face.

[273] Evodia specifically works on the liver channel and, at the same time, enters the spleen and stomach. It has similar actions to those of Cornus and, therefore, mainly treats a similar spectrum of diseases. Because it is able to precipitate the qi, it is a good remedy for qi counterflow, abdominal urgency, intestinal wind, and hemorrhoids. Li Gao said:

(continued...)

warms the center, precipitates the qi, relieves pain, cough and counterflow, and cold and heat. It eliminates dampness and blood impediment, expels wind evil, and opens the interstices. Its root (Radix Evodiae Rutecarpae) kills the three [kinds of] worms. Its other name is *Yi* (Cooked Yam). It grows in rivers and valleys.

Qin Pi (Cortex Fraxini)[274] is sour. It is nontoxic, mainly treating wind cold damp impediment and continual cold qi. It eliminates fever and green-blue and white screen in the eye. Protracted taking may keep the head [hair] from becoming white and make the body light. It grows in rivers and valleys.

Zhi Zi (Fructus Gardeniae Jasminoidis)[275] is bitter and cold. It mainly treats evil qi in the five internals [*i.e.*, five viscera], heat qi in the stomach,

---

[273](...continued)

When turbid yin cannot descend and reversal qi counterflows upward, obstructed diaphragm with [chest] distention and fullness will arise. Then, but for Evodia, it cannot be cured. In addition, such conditions as desire to vomit after eating which is due to liver cold assaulting the stomach, stomach cold glomus, fullness and dysphagia-occlusion are all also its indications. What's more, Evodia is effective for precipitating blood stasis in the lower abdomen and postpartum retained blood.

Evodia is also good at expelling wind evils and opening the interstices. Therefore, it is able to treat fire sores in children, *jue yin* headache, wind papules, and lacquer sores.

[274] Fraxinus levels the liver and, therefore, is a good medicinal for eye diseases and heat dysentery. In modern prescriptions, it is sometimes used to treat scanty semen in males and vaginal discharge in females. However, it is seldom used for the other indications given in the text.

[275] Gardenia is a medicinal for the heart, liver, and stomach. It is able to penetrate the qi and blood, particularly the blood. Because it is bitter and cold, it drains heat from the heart and lungs to resolve fire depression of the triple burner. Therefore, conditions like reversal heat heart pain are resolved. Even more remakable is its ability to cure heart vexation and anguish, insomnia, and various categories of jaundice. It should be noted that nearly all empirically proven formulas for jaundice contain Gardenia.

red boils on the face, drinker's nose, white *lai* and red *lai*[266] and sores. Its other name is *Mu Dan* (Wood Cinnabar). It grows in rivers and valleys.

He Huan (Cortex Albizziae Julibrissinis) is sweet and balanced. It mainly quiets the five viscera, harmonizes the heart and will [*i.e.*, the emotions], and makes one happy and worry-free. Protracted taking may make the body light, brighten the eyes, and [put one in a contented frame of mind as if one had] acquired whatever one desired. It grows in the mountains and valleys of Yi Zhou.[276]

Qin Jiao (Pericarpium Zanthoxyli Peperiti)[277] is acrid and warm. It mainly treats wind evil qi, warms the center, eliminates cold impediment, fortifies the teeth, promotes the growth of hair, and brightens the eyes. Protracted taking may make the body light, render a good facial complexion, slow aging, prolong life, and enable one to communicate with spirits. It grows in rivers and valleys.

---

[276] *I.e.*, an area around present-day Chengdu, Sichuan Province

[277] *Qin Jiao* (Zanthoxylum Peperitum) belongs to the same genus as *Chuan Jiao* or *Shu Jiao* (Zanthoxylum Bungeanum). However, its fruit is bigger. As medicinals, these two have the same actions. This medicinal is acrid and hot and is purely yang in nature. Therefore, it is able to supplement the life gate fire to treat kidney qi upward counterflow, yang debility frequent urination, night sweats, and seminal efflux. In addition, it fortifies the teeth and frees the flow of the channels. Moreover, it is capable of promoting sweating and effusing cold. As such, it is used to treat cold damage cough and throat impediment. Zanthoxylum is inclined to enter the spleen, and its other action is to dry dampness and eliminate cold. For that reason, it is often used to disperse food, eliminate distention, and relieve heart and abdominal cold pain, vomiting, dysentery, phlegm rheum, and water swelling. For the above indications, the pericarp (Pericarpium) is used. However, the seed (Semen) is also a commonly used medicinal. It is called *Jiao Mu*. It is particularly good for moving water to treat swelling.

Zi Wei **(Flos Campsitis Grandiflorae)**[278] is sour and slightly cold. It mainly treats women's breast-feeding and postpartum illnesses, flooding, concretions and conglomerations, blood block, cold and heat, and languor and emaciation. It nourishes the fetus. It grows in rivers and valleys.

Wu Yi **(Semen Fermentatum Ulmi Macrocarpae)**[279] is acrid. It mainly treats evil qi in the five internals, dissipates excessive moving toxins in the skin, flesh, and bone joints,[280] removes the three [kinds of] worms, and transforms food. Its other name is *Wu Gu* (Wu Mushroom). Yet another name is *Dian Tang* (Starch Sugar). It grows in rivers and valleys.

Sang Gen Bai Pi **(Cortex Radicis Mori Albi)**[281] is sweet and cold. It mainly treats damaged center, the five taxations and six extremes, languor and emaciation, flooding, and expiry of the pulse. It supplements vacuity and boosts the qi. Its leaf [Folium Mori Albi][282] eliminates cold and heat and promotes sweating.

---

[278] This medicinal is able to remove hidden fire in the blood and break the blood to eliminate stasis. Therefore, it is an important medicinal for diseases in women. As such, however, this medicinal should be able to induce abortion rather than to nourish the fetus as is said in the text. In fact, an alternative name for this medicinal is *Duo Tai Hua*, Falling Fetus Flower.

[279] In modern clinical practice, this medicinal is an important one for parasites and cold large intestinal efflux. The latter is a kind of diarrhea.

[280] This phrase is confusing. Based on references in related literature, it may mean wind in the muscles, skin, and joints causing a feeling as if worms were moving within them, *i.e.*, formication.

[281] Mulberry Root Bark drains fire qi by moving water qi from the lungs through urination. Therefore, it treats effulgent heat, cough followed by panting, swollen face, generalized fever, and inhibited urination. Some of its actions listed in the text, for example, recuperating a damaged center and supplementing the five taxations, should be ascribed to the fruit (*Sang Zhi*, Fructus Mori Albi) rather than the root bark.

[282] Mulberry Leaves cool the blood, eliminate wind, dry dampness, blacken the beard and head hair, and brighten the eyes. They are good for eye diseases when used in the form of a decoction to wash the eyes. In addition, they are able to stop night sweats.

101

Sang Er **(Fructificatio Aurilae Judae** growing on the mulberry) is black. It mainly cures women's leaking, red and white vaginal discharge, blood diseases, concretions and conglomerations, accumulations and gatherings, abdominal pain, yin and yang [disharmony], cold and heat, and infertility.

The five [kinds of] *Mu Er* **(Fructificatio Aurilae Judae)**,[283] called *Lin* (Windowsill), boost the qi, make one free from hunger and the body light, and fortify the will [*i.e.*, the mind]. They grow in mountains and valleys.

---

[283] The five *Mu Er* or Wood Ears include Fructuficatio Ariculae Judae growing on logs of mulberry, paper mulberry, Chinese scholartree, elm, and willow.

Woods: Inferior Class

Song Luo **(Herba Usneae Longissimae)**[284] is bitter and balanced. It mainly treats indignation and anger evil qi and relieves vacuity sweating, head wind, and, in females, genital cold, swelling, and pain. Its other name is *Nu Luo* (Female Creeper). It grows in mountains and valleys.

Wu Jia **(Cortex Radicis Acanthopanacis Gracilistyli)**[285] is acrid and warm. It mainly treats heart and abdominal mounting qi and abdominal pain. It boosts the qi and heals limpness, enabling the [limp] child to walk instantly. [It also treats] flat abscesses, sores, and genital erosion. Its other name is *Chai Qi* (Jackal Lacquer).

Zhu Ling **(Sclerotium Polypori Umbellati)**[286] is sweet and balanced. It mainly treats malaria, resolves toxins, *gu* toxins, *gu* influx, and ill matters and disinhibits the water passageways. Protracted taking may make the body light and slow aging. Its other name is *Jia Zhu Shi* (Pig Droppings).

---

[284] This medicinal also treats cold and heat, removes phlegm from the chest, and cures head sores. However, it is no longer used.

[285] This medicinal's current name is *Wu Jia Pi*. Acanthopanax Root Bark normalizes the qi and transforms phlegm, boosts the qi and fortifies the bone, expels wind and overcomes dampness. It treats vacuity taxation, hypertonicity of the sinews, impotence, genital damp itch in females, and weak feet in children. In modern prescriptions, it is used as an important medicinal for expelling wind dampness and fortifying the sinews and bones.

[286] Polyporus opens the interstices, promotes sweating, and disinhibits urination. Its actions are similar to those of Poria, but it does not supplement vacuity. Therefore, its indications are narrower. It treats cold damage, damp phlegm, intense fever, a burning sensation in the heart, wasting thirst, swelling, distention, strangury, turbidity, malaria, and dysentery.

It grows in mountains and valleys.

Bai Ji (**Spina Zizyphi Spinosae**)[287] is acrid and cold. It mainly treats heart and abdominal pain, welling abscesses, swellings, and suppuration. It relieves pain. Its other name is *Ji Zhen* (Spinous Needle). It grows in rivers and valleys.

Wei Mao (**Suberalatum Euonymi Alatae**)[288] is bitter and cold. It is nontoxic, mainly treating flooding and [vaginal] bleeding in females, abdominal fullness, and sweating. It eliminates evils, killing ghost toxins and *gu* influx. Its other name is *Gui Jian* (Ghost Arrow).

Huang Huan[289] is bitter. It is toxic, mainly treating *gu* toxins, demonic influx, and ghost obssession, and evil qi in the viscera. It eliminates cough and counterflow and cold and heat. Its other name is *Ling Quan* (Mound Spring). Yet another name is *Da Jiu* (Great Accomplishment). It grows in mountains and valleys.

Shi Nan Cao (**Folium Photiniae Serrulatae**)[290] is acrid and balanced. It

---

[287] This medicinal went out of use in the Song dynasty.

[288] The current name of this medicinal is *Gui Jian*. It breaks the blood and frees the channels (or menses), kills worms and expels ill matters. It may be used to treat postpartum vanquished blood and sudden heart pain. In modern clinical practice, however, it is seldom if ever employed. In some versions, this medicinal is categorized as being in the middle class.

[289] This medicinal has long been out of use and its identity cannot now be determined.

[290] This medicinal mainly treats kidney vacuity foot weakness and wind impediment. It was said that women should not take it. Otherwise they might become lustful after men. There was also another warning that anyone who took it might suffer yin wilting (one of whose manifestation is impotence). Li Shi-zhen rejected these statements, saying:

...this medicinal may fortify the kidneys. Some people take it for the purpose of living a libertine life, thus contracting wilting and weakness.

(continued...)

mainly nourishes the kidney qi, damaged internal damage, and debilitated yin and benefits the sinews, bones, skin, and hair. Its seed [Semen Photiniae Serrulatae] kills *gu* toxins, breaks accumulations and gatherings, and expels wind impediment. Its other name is *Gui Mu* (Ghost Eye). It grows in mountains and valleys.

Ba Dou (**Semen Crotonis Tiglii**)[291] is acrid and warm. It is toxic. It mainly treats cold damage, warm malaria, and cold and heat. It breaks concretions and conglomerations, bindings and gatherings, hard accumulations, lodged rheum, and phlegm aggregation as well as [relieves] enlarged abdomen water distention. It flushes the five viscera and six bowels, opens and unblocks blocks and congestions, disinhibits the passageways of water and grain, removes malign flesh, eliminates ghost toxins, *gu* influx, and evil matters, and kills worms and fish. Its other name is *Ba Jiao* (Ba Pepper). It grows in rivers and valleys.

---

[290](...continued)

In other words, the wilting and weakness was not a direct result of the use of this medicinal but rather the effect of excessive sexual activity resulting in debility detriment. Nowadays, it is an important medicinal in the treatment of threatened miscarriage.

[291] Croton Seeds overcome cold and expel water. This text provides an exhaustive list of their indications, including phlegm aggregation, blood conglomerations, qi glomus, food accumulations, enlarged abdomen, water swelling, diarrhea, dysentery, deviated mouth, deafness, toothache, throat impediment, sores, and snake and scorpion toxins. In addition, it kills parasites, induces abortion, and heals decayed flesh. It is very strong in precipitation and breaking block. There are many formulas composed of Croton Seeds for various emergency cases. For example, for the block pattern of wind stroke, which manifests as abdominal fullness, urinary and fecal stoppage, clouded spirit, clenched jaws, and phlegm rales in the throat, there is *Duo Ming San* (Snatch Life Back Powder) composed of *Ba Dou* (Semen Crotonis), *Ban Xia* (Rhizoma Pinelliae Ternatae), *Ting Li* (Semen Lepidii Seu Descurainiae), and *Nan Xing* (Rhizoma Arisaematis). It is said that the condition will be relieved once phlegm is ejected after this formula is taken. For another example, when there is fulminant heart and abdominal pain and fullness, clenched jaw, and urinary and fecal stoppage, *San Wu Bei Ji Fang* (Three Materials Emergency Formula) is quite effective. This formula is composed of *Ba Dou* (Semen Crotonis), *Jie Geng* (Radix Platycodi Grandiflori), *Bei Mu* (Bulbus Fritillariae), and *Jiang* (Rhizoma Zingiberis).

105

Shu Jiao (Pericarpium Zanthoxyli Bungeani)[292] is acrid and warm. It mainly treats evil qi, cough and counterflow, warms the center, expels [cold dampness in] the bones and joints, skin and the flesh, [removes] dead muscles and cold damp impediment pain, and precipitates the qi. Protracted taking may keep the head [hair] from becoming white, make the body light, and increase the life span. It grows in rivers and valleys.

Mang Cao (Folium Illicii Anisati)[293] is acrid and warm. It mainly treats head wind, welling abscesses, swellings, mammary abscesses, and mounting conglomeration. It eliminates binding qi, itchy scabs, flat abscesses, and sores and kills worms and fish. It grows in mountains and valleys.

Yu He (Semen Pruni)[294] is sour and balanced. It mainly treats enlarged abdomen water swelling and puffy swelling of the face, eyes, and limbs. It disinhibits urination and the water passageways. Its root [Radix Pruni] mainly treats broken teeth with swollen [gums] and tooth decay and

---

[292] This medicinal has the same actions as *Qin Jiao*. See *Qin Jiao* in the Middle Class of Woods above. It is used mainly for warming the stomach, dispersing food, and supplementing the true fire of the life gate.

[293] This medicinal is drastic and toxic and, therefore, is seldom administered orally. In modern prescriptions, it is only applied externally and even then but seldom.

[294] The current name is *Yu Li Ren*. This medicinal precipitates the qi, breaks aggregations and moves water, and hence is an important medicinal for water swelling. According to a proven formula, smashed Prune Seed in combination with *Yi Yi Ren* (Semen Coicis Lachryma-jobi) is able to treat foot qi puffy swelling, heart and abdominal fullness, urinary and fecal stoppage, and rapid panting. Foot qi is a syndrome of water swelling starting from the feet and gradually extending upwards. It is usually complicated by numbness of the feet and, in the advanced stage, cardiac and mental disorders such as delirious speech and clouded spirit.

fortifies the teeth. *Shu Li* (Cortex Rhamni Pershianae)[295] mainly treats cold and heat, scrofulas, and sores. [Semen Pruni] is also called *Jue Li* (Tripod Plum). It grows in rivers and valleys.

Luan Hua (Flos Koelreuteriae Paniculatae) is bitter and cold. It mainly treats eye pain, tearing, and injured canthi and disperses eye swelling. It grows in rivers and valleys.

Man Jiao **(Pericarpium Zanthoxyli Simulantis)**[296] is bitter and warm. It mainly treats wind cold damp impediment and joint-running pain and eliminates reversal qi in the limbs and pain in the knees. Its other name is *Shi Jiao* (Pig Pepper). It grows in rivers and valleys.

Lei Wan **(Sclerotium Omphaliae Lapidescentis)**[297] is bitter and cold. It mainly kills the three [kinds of] worms, expels toxic qi and heat in the stomach, and benefits males but not females. It can make paste to eliminate the hundreds of diseases in children. It grows in mountains and valleys.

Sou Shu **(Semen Deutziae Scabrae)**[298] is acrid and cold. It mainly treats generalized and skin fever, eliminates evil qi, and stops enuresis. It can be used to make bathwater. It grows in rivers and valleys.

---

[295] *Shu Li* (Cortex Rhamni Purshianae) is a different species from *Yu Li* (Prunus Japonicae). But for some reason during long circulation, it is now included in this passage. One should also note that, as a medicinal, it is its bark rather than its seed that is used.

[296] This medicinal belongs to a species of Zanthoxylum which is a large family. Its definite identity is still an open issue.

[297] Omphalia is now used specifically for parasites. The statement in the text that this medicinal brings benefit to males but does harm to females has been a controversial issue. One reasonable interpretation is that it dredges and disinhibits the qi in males but does not do so in females.

[298] The primary actions of this medicinal include disinhibiting the water passageways, eliminating heat in the stomach, and precipitating the qi.

107

Yao Shi Gen (**Radix Fritillariae**)²⁹⁹ is acrid and warm. It mainly treats evil qi and various impediment aching pain, mends expiry and damage, and supplements the bone marrow. Its other name is *Lian Mu* (Linking Wood). It grows in mountains and valleys.

Zao Jia (**Fructus Gleditschiae Chinensis**)³⁰⁰ is acrid, salty, and warm. It mainly treats wind impediment, dead muscles, evil qi, head wind, and tearing. It disinhibits the nine orifices and kills spiritual matters. It grows in rivers and valleys.

Lian Shi (**Fructus Meliae Toosendan**)³⁰¹ is bitter and cold. It mainly treats warm disease, cold damage, great fever, vexation, and mania. It kills the three [kinds of] worms, [heals] scab sores, and disinhibits urination and the water passageways. It grows in mountains and valleys.

Liu Hua (**Flos Salicis Babylonicae**) is bitter and cold. It mainly treats wind water, jaundice, and heat black complexion of the face. Its leaves [Folium Salicis Babylonicae] mainly treat scab sores in horses. Its fruit [Fructus Salicis Babylonicae] mainly treats open welling abscesses and expels pus

---

²⁹⁹ Concerning the true identity of this medicinal, there is not yet consensus. One problem is certain. If the plant is Fritillaria, the medicinal should be its bulb rather than the root as the Chinese word *gen* suggests.

³⁰⁰ Gleditsia is a good emetic. It provokes sneezing, disperses wind phlegm, dissipates swelling, kills worms, and lubricates the large intestine, *i.e.*, removes constipation. Therefore, it is often used to treat the conditions of loss of consciousness and inability to speak. Externally applied, it can treat impediment pain, welling and flat abscesses, sores, and swellings. However, it should not be used in pregnant women without warrant.

³⁰¹ Melia Toosendan Fruit drains heat in the bladder and small intestine and downbears fire in the pericardium. Therefore, it treats distention and pain in the cardiac region and abdomen. Besides what is explained in the text, it is a good medicinal for mounting due to cold. However, for parasites, the root bark of the plant, which is called *Ku Lian Gen Pi* (Cortex Radicis Meliae Azardachis) is now used instead of the fruit.

and [decayed] blood. Its other name is *Liu Xu* (Willow Fiber). It grows in the rivers and swamps of Lang Ya.[302]

Tong Ye (**Folium Sterculiae Platanifoliae**) is bitter and cold. It mainly treats malign and eroding sores fixed to yin [*i.e.*, deep-seated sores]. Its bark [Cortex Sterculiae] mainly treats the five kinds of hemorrhoids and kills the three [kinds of] worms. Its flower [Flos Sterculiae] can be applied to sores in pigs. If it is fed to pigs, the pigs may grow four times larger. [This medicinal] grows in mountains and valleys.

Zi Bai Pi (**Cortex Catalpae Bungei**) is bitter and cold. It mainly treats heat and kills the three [kinds of] worms. Its flower and leaf [Flos Et Folium Catalpae] can be pounded and [then] applied to sores in pigs. If they are fed to pigs, the pigs may grow four times larger. It grows in mountains and valleys.

Huai Mu (**Old Decayed Wood**)[303] is bitter and balanced. It is nontoxic, mainly treating enduring cough with qi ascent, damaged center, vacuity, languor, and, in females, genital erosion, leaking, and red and white vaginal discharge. Its other name is *Bai Sui Cheng Zhong Mu* (Wood in the Hundred Year Old Town). It is produced in plains and swamps.

---

[302] *I.e.*, present-day Shandong Peninsula

[303] This medicinal is made from decayed wood as, for example, poles and stakes found in old buildings.

Ben Cao Jing
Book Three

Animals: Superior Class

Fa Bei (Crinis Humanis)[304] is bitter and warm. It mainly treats the five [kinds of] dribbling urinary block and block and repulsion. It disinhibits urination and the water passageways and cures epilepsy in children and tetany in adults. It may return to divinity again.[305]

---

[304] The current name is *Xue Yu* (Blood Surplus) or *Ren Fa* (Human Hair). This medicinal is able to disperse stasis and disinhibit urination and defecation. In modern prescriptions, *Xue Yu Tan* (Crinis Carbonisatus) is often used to cure disorders related to the blood, for example, tongue bleeding, nosebleeding, blood strangury, and blood dysentery.

[305] In ancient times, head hair was deemed a sacred part of the body. Confucius, for example, said, "One's hair is gifted from one's parents." Hence, it should be taken good care of. This sentence is a little confusing. It might imply that when hair was cut, which was a violation of the tenet that hair should be protected as well as one's life, it might grow again as a holy substance.

Long Gu (Os Draconis)[306] is sweet and balanced. It mainly treats heart and abdominal demonic influx, spiritual matters, old ghosts, cough and counterflow, diarrhea and dysentery of pus and blood, in females, leaking, concretions and conglomerations, hardness and binding, and, in children, heat qi and fright epilepsy. *Long Chi* (Dens Draconis)[307] mainly treats children and adults alike of epilepsy, madness, maniac running about, binding qi below the heart, inability to catch one's breath, and various [kinds of] tetany. It kills spiritual matters. Protracted taking may make the body light, enable one to communicate with the spirit light, and lenghten one's life span. It is produced in mountains and valleys.

Niu Huang (Calculus Bovis)[308] is bitter and balanced. It mainly treats fright epilepsy, cold and heat, and intense heat, mania, and tetany. It eliminates evils and dispels ghosts. The tip of the cow horn [Apex Cornu Bovis]

---

[306] Dragon Bone is, as a matter of fact, fossilized animal bones, most often deer bone. It is sweet and astringent in flavor and slightly cold of qi. It astringes the intestines, boosts the kidneys, secures the essence, stops sweating, quiets the ethereal soul, and stabilizes the corporeal soul. It is often prescribed to treat dream-fraught sleep, fright epilepsy, withdrawal and mania, blood ejection, nosebleed, flooding, vaginal discharge, seminal emission, prolapse of the rectum, etc. Chen Xiu-yuan said:

> Dragon Bone is able to astringe fire and quiet the spirit, dispel phlegm and downbear counterflow. Therefore, it is a miraculous medicinal for fright epilepsy, madness, and tetany.

[307] *Long Chi* (Dens Draconis) is actually fossilized mastodon teeth, Palaeoloxodon Nomadicus or Archidoskodon Planifronis. It is cold of qi and its actions are similar to those of *Long Gu* (Os Draconis). Besides the indications listed in the text, it has a good effect on heart pain.

[308] This medicinal clears the heart and resolves heat, disinhibits phlegm and suppresses fright. It is often used to treat fright epilepsy and wind stroke of the viscera which is a critical condition manifesting mainly as sudden collapse with inability to recognize people. There are two patterns of visceral stroke—block and desertion. The block pattern is characterized by clenched jaws, urinary and fecal stoppage, and hypertonicity. The desertion pattern is featured by faint breathing, sweating, urinary and fecal incontinence, and an expiring pulse. Cow Bezoar is very effective for both patterns of visceral stroke. However, it should not be used for channel stroke.

112

precipitates blocked blood and blood stasis causing aching pain and, in females, [treats] vaginal discharge and [uterine] bleeding. The marrow [Medulla Bovis] supplements the center and replenishes the bone marrow. Protracted taking may lengthen the life span. The bile [Fel Bovis] can make pills. [Cows] grow in the plains and swamps.

She Xiang (Secretio Moschi)[309] is acrid and warm. It mainly keeps off malign qi, kills ghosts and spiritual matters, [cures] warm malaria, *gu* toxins, epilepsy, and tetany, and removes the three [kinds of] worms. Protracted taking may eliminate evils to prevent depressive ghost dreams in sleep. It is produced in rivers and valleys.

Xiong Zhi (Adeps Ursi)[310] is sweet and slightly cold. It mainly treats wind impediment, insensitivity, hypertonicity of the sinews, accumulations and gatherings in the five viscera and abdomen, cold and heat, languor and emaciation, head sores, bald white scalp sores, and black patches and boils on the face. Protracted taking may fortify the will and make one free from hunger and the body light. It is produced in mountains and valleys.

---

[309] Musk opens the vessel network and frees the orifices and, therefore, is good for wind stroke, phlegm reversal, fright epilepsy, and heart and abdominal distention, pain, glomus and fullness. This medicinal has a wide range of indications. For example, *Tong Qiao Huo Xue Tang* (Free the Orifices & Quicken the Blood Decoction) with Musk as a main ingredient is very effective for taxation vacuity, baldness, drinker's nose, and *gan* in children which manifests mainly as dyspepsia, increasing emaciation, and enlarged abdomen.

[310] This is the fat growing in the back of the bear. However, it is seldom used nowadays. Instead *Xiong Dan* (Fel Ursi), which is able to cool the heart and level the liver, is often prescribed to treat fright epilepsy, various hemorrhoids, *gan* in children, malign sores, and jaundice. In addition, because it levels the liver, it is capable of brightening the eyes.

113

Bai Jiao (Gelatinum Cornu Cervi)[311] is sweet and balanced. It mainly treats damaged center, taxation expiry, lumbago, and languor and emaciation. It supplements the center and boosts the qi. In females, [it treats] blood block infertility, relieves [abdominal] pain, and quiets the fetus. Protracted taking may make the body light and prolong life. Its other name is *Lu Jiao Jiao* (Deer Horn Glue).

E Jiao (Gelatinum Corii Asini)[312] is sweet and balanced. It mainly treats heart and abdominal internal flooding, extreme taxation, chills as in malaria, pain in the lumbus and abdomen, and aching pain in the limbs. In females, it precipitates the blood and quiets the fetus. Protracted taking may make the body light and boost the qi. Its other name is *Chuan Zhi Jiao* (Passing Glue).

Dan Xiong Ji (Gallus Rubrus Masculinus)[313] is sweet and slightly warm. It mainly treats flooding and leaking and red and white vaginal discharge

---

[311] The current name is *Lu Jiao Jiao*. This medicinal is sweet in flavor and warm of qi. It supplements the essence and blood and fortifies the sinews and bones. It is often prescribed to treat kidney vacuity cold, taxation damage, and aching pain in the limbs. Because it supplements very strongly, it is only appropriate for fire debility conditions with a deep and fine pulse.

[312] Ass Hide Glue is able to clear the lungs and nourish the liver, enrich the kidneys and supplement yin. It is an important medicinal for supplementing the blood and is often prescribed to treat various conditions related to the blood, for example, blood ejection, hemorrhoids, hemafecia, menstrual irregularities, flooding, and stirring fetus. In his *Ming Yi Bie Lu* (*Collected Extracts from Distinguished Physicians*), Tao Hong-jing said, Ass Hide Glue's "indications include lower abdominal pain in males, vacuity taxation, insufficient yin qi, aching feet with inability to stand up for long, and nourishing the liver qi."

[313] This medicinal is red, male Chicken. However, since the end of the Han dynasty, the sex and color of chickens have not been taken into account when they are used as a medicinal. Generally speaking, Chicken is able to supplement vacuity and warm the center. In this passage, several different parts of the chicken are discussed as separate medicinals. In modern prescriptions, however, only *Bi Zhi* or *Ji Nei Jin* (Endothelium Corneum Gigeriae Galli) in modern terms is commonly used as a medicinal. Able to promote digestion, it is a remedy for food damage, stomach reflux, diarrhea, and dysentery. Besides, it treats frequent urination, enuresis, hematuria, flooding, and vaginal discharge.

in females. It supplements vacuity, warms the center, frees the spirit, kills toxins, and wards off ill matters. The head [Caput Galli] mainly kills ghosts. The fat [Adeps Galli] mainly treats deafness. The intestines [Intestinus Galli] mainly treats enuresis. The gizzard [Gigeria Galli] with its yellow membrane mainly treats diarrhea and dysentery. The white of the chicken's dropping mainly treats wasting thirst, cold damage, and cold and heat. The feathers [Pluma Galli] mainly precipitate blood block. The egg [Ovum Galli] eliminates fire heat sores, epilepsy, and tetany. It is capable of making the divine thing, amber. Fleas on chickens[314] may fatten pigs. [Chickens] grow in the plains and swamps.

Yan Fang (Adeps Anas)[315] is sweet and balanced. It is nontoxic, mainly treating wind hypertonicity, hemilateral withering, and inhibited qi. Protracted taking may boost the qi, make one free from hunger and the body light, and slow aging. Its other name is *Wu Fang* (Wild Duck Fat). [Ducks] grow in pools and swamps.

Shi Mi (Mel)[316] is sweet and balanced. It mainly treats heart and abdominal evil qi, all fright epilepsy, and tetany. It quiets the five viscera when they sustain various insufficiencies, boosts the qi, supplements the center, relieves pain, and resolves toxins. It eliminates multitudes of diseases and harmonizes hundreds of medicinals. Protracted taking may fortify the will, make the body light and free from hunger, and prevent senility. It is produced in mountains and valleys.

---

[314] The identity of this medicinal is questionable.

[315] This bird is either the domesticated or wild duck. Nowadays, it is seldom used as a medicinal.

[316] Honey moistens dryness, resolves various toxins, relieves various kinds of pain, frees the flow of the triple burner, and harmonizes the constructive and defensive. It is often prescribed to suppress cough, cure dysentery, and brighten the eyes. Besides the indications listed in the text, it may render the face brilliant.

Mi La (**Cera Alba**)[317] is sweet and slightly warm. It mainly treats dysentery with pus and blood, supplements the center, and mends expiry and damage and incised wounds. It boosts the qi, makes one free from hunger, and slows aging. It is produced in mountains and valleys.

Feng Zi (**Larva Apis Ceranae**)[318] is sweet and balanced. It mainly treats head wind, eliminates *gu* toxins, and supplements vacuity and languor and damaged center. Protracted taking may make one have a brilliant, lovely facial complexion and prevent senility. *Da Huang Feng Zi* (Larva Vespae) mainly treats heart and abdominal distention, fullness and pain. It may make the body light and boost the qi. *Tu Feng Zi* (Larva Scoliae) mainly treats welling abscesses and swellings. Another name [for Larva Scoliae] is *Fei Ling* (Lonely Fly). They grow in mountains and valleys.

---

[317] In modern prescriptions, wax is seldom administered orally except when it is used as a coating of pills. It is sometimes applied externally to treat frostbite.

[318] Tao Hong-jing said, "It mainly treats heart and abdominal pain, vomiting of the five kinds of worms in the abdomen in both adults and children, and yellowing of the face and eyes." Zhao Xue-min (1719-1805 CE) said in his *Ben Cao Gang Mu Shi Yi* (*A Supplement to the Outlines of Materia Medica*), "Bee Chrysalis mainly treats cinnabar toxins, wind papules, lodging heat in the abdomen, and inhibited urination and defecation...It treats vaginal discharge and promotes lactation in women."

Mu Li (**Concha Ostreae**)[319] is salty and balanced. It mainly treats cold damage, cold and heat, warm malaria with chills, and fright, indignation and anger qi. It eliminates tuggings and slackenings, mouse fistulas, and, in females, red and white vaginal discharge. Protracted taking may fortify the bone joints, kill evil ghosts, and prolong life. Its other name is *Li He* (Oyster Shell). It grows in pools and swamps.

---

[319] Oyster Shell is able to soften hardness and transform phlegm, astringe and clear heat, and disinhibit dampness. For that reason, it is a good medicinal for scrofulas, nodes, concretions and conglomerations, seminal emission, flooding, cough, copious sweating, vacuity taxation, vexatious fever, and intestinal efflux. Wang Hao-gu said:

Conducted by Bupleurum, it may remove hardness in the rib-side region. Conducted by Tea, it disperses nodes in the neck. Conducted by Rhubarb, it disperses swelling in the thigh. With Rehmannia as its envoy, it boosts and astringes the essence and stops frequent urination. With Fritillaria as its envoy, it disperses accumulations and binding.

Chen Nian-zu gave an interesting account of the mechanism of the actions of Oyster Shell when he said:

This substance is bestowed with the nature of both metal and water. When cold damage transmits into the *shao yang* channel, it gives rise to alternating cold and heat. This falls within the indications [of Oyster Shell]. Underlying [these indications] is the qi of metal and water which is able to stop the wandering wood fire. Warm malaria is a kind of malaria where there is merely heat without cold. There is a heat disease of the *yang ming* channel, which manifests slight cold in the back or rather aversion to cold. [Now] fire is inclined to start up but cannot reach the channel. The reason why Oyster Shell is used as a principal [medicinal for those cases] is to exploit its metal qi [or autumn astringing qi] to resolve the intense summerheat [meaning fire here]. Fright, indignation, and anger qi is governed by the heart but starts in the liver. Oyster Shell is balanced in terms of qi. This enables it to exert the action of metal so as to restrain wood. Its salty flavor enables it to exert the action of water so as to overwhelm fire. Tuggings and slackenings are a liver illness, and mouse fistulas are a fire depression disease of the triple burner and gallbladder channel. The balanced [qi] of Oyster Shell is able to restrain wind cold and overwhelm fire. Saltiness is able to soften hardness...

Li Yu Dan (**Fel Cyprini Carpionis**)[320] is bitter and cold. It mainly treats eye heat, redness, pain, and clear-eye blindness. It brightens the eyes. Protracted taking may strengthen and boost the will and qi. [Carp] grow in pools and swamps.

Feng Yu (**Ophiocephalus Argus**) is sweet and cold. It mainly treats damp impediment and puffy swelling of the face and eyes. It precipitates great water.[321] Its other name is *Tong Yu* (Copper Fish). It grows in pools and swamps.

---

[320] Carp Gall may treat swollen throat and throat impediment besides what is explained in the text. It is said in the *Tu Jing (Illustrated [Materia Medica] Classic)* by Su Jing of the Tang dynasty that the gall, flesh, bone, and teeth of the carp can all be used as medicinals. The flesh disinhibits urination and treats foot qi water swelling, night sweats, and jaundice. The bone ash treats bones stuck in the throat. Nowadays, however, carp gall seems to be used the least often.

[321] Great water means serious edema.

Animals: Middle Class

Xi Jiao (Cornu Rhinocerotis)[322] is bitter and cold. It mainly treats the hundreds of toxins, *gu* influx, evil ghosts, and miasmic qi, kills Liphooking,[323] *zhen* feather,[324] and snake toxins, eliminates evils, and prevents confusion and oppressive ghost dreams. Protracted taking may make the body light. It is produced in rivers and valleys.

---

[322] The actions of Rhinoceros Horn include cooling the heart and draining the liver, clearing stomach heat, expelling wind and disinhibiting phlegm, and resolving toxins. Besides the indications in the text, this medicinal is often prescribed for cold damage, jaundice, macular eruptions, blood ejection, hemafecia, blood amassment delirium and mania, fright wind, and pox sores. Rhinoceros Horn is a wonderful medicinal for clearing heat and cooling the blood. The famous *Xi Jiao Di Huang Tang* (Rhinoceros Horn & Rehmannia Decoction), for example, is a very effective formula for heat damage giving rise to blood ejection, nosebleed, hemafecia, and, in females, flooding and red strangury. Used alone, Rhinoceros Horn is also able to treat fright epilepsy in children, loss of consciousness, and food poisoning. However, because this medicinal is from a severely endangered species, it should no longer be used. Instead, one can substitute Cornu Bubali (*Shui Niu Jiao*, Water Buffalo Horn) in larger doses.

[323] This is the name of a fatally poisonous herb. However, here, it refers to all such poisonous herbs in general. It is said that after even one bite of this herb, the person will collapse on the spot as if their mouth were hooked by the herb.

[324] The *zhen* was a legendary bird which was believed to be so poisonous that one would be killed the moment one drank a drop of wine in which a feather of the *zhen* had been dipped.

Ling Yang Jiao (Cornu Antelopis Saiga-tatarici)[325] is salty and cold. It mainly brightens the eyes, boosts the qi, lifts yin, removes malign blood and downpour diarrhea, wards off *gu* toxins, vicious ghosts, and ill matters, quiets the heart qi, and prevents oppressive ghost dreams. Protracted taking may fortify the sinews and bones and make the body light. It is produced in rivers and valleys.

Gu Yang Jiao (Cornu Caprae Seu Ovis)[326] is salty and warm. It mainly treats clear-eye blindness, brightens the eyes, kills scab worms, checks cold diarrhea, keeps off malign ghosts and tigers and wolves,[327] and suppresses fright palpitations. Protracted taking may quiet the heart, boost the qi, and make the body light. It is produced in rivers and valleys.

Bai Ma Jing (Penis Equi Caballi Albi) is salty and balanced. It mainly treats damaged center, expired pulse, and impotence. It fortifies the will, boosts the qi, promotes the growth of the muscles and flesh, makes one fat and strong, and makes pregnancy possible. The eyes [Oculus Equi Caballi] mainly treat fright epilepsy, abdominal fullness, and malaria disease. The

---

[325] This medicinal is mainly for troubles related to the liver and heart channels. It precipitates the qi and downbears fire, resolves toxins and keeps off evils, dissipates the blood and disperses stasis. It mainly treats mania, fright epilepsy, hypertonicity, bone pain, mounting qi, and eye screen. Used singly, it may treat dysphagia-occlusion and heat toxins hemafecia. It can also hasten delivery. If administered after being burnt, it treats heart vexation and fullness due to blood and qi counterflow, postpartum inability to recognize people, and dysentery in children. When used in combination with other medicinals, it has an even wider range of curative effects.

[326] In his *Ming Yi Bie Lu*, Tao Hong-jing said, "It cures bound qi in the hundreds of joints, wind headache, *gu* toxins, blood ejection, and postpartum pain in women..." Goat Horn is usually used singly. It is seldom combined with other medicinals. Stir-fried Goat Horn dust, for example, can treat wind giving rise to heart vexation, abstraction, and abdominal pain or temporary faintness. Mixed with egg whites, the horn ash can be applied to sudden red macular eruptions.

[327] In the literature, we can find descriptions of how to burn Goat Horn to ward off snakes with the smoke. However, the method of using this horn to keep away beasts is unknown.

suspended hoof [328] mainly treats fright evils, tuggings and slackenings, and difficult lactation. It keeps off malign qi, ghost toxins, *gu* influx, and ill matters. [Horses] grow in plains and swamps.

Gou Yin Jing **(Penis Canis)** is salty and balanced. It mainly treats damaged center and impotence, causes intense heat and pregnancy, and eliminates the 12 diseases of vaginal discharge[329] in females. The gall [Fel Canis][330] brightens the eyes. Another name [of the dog's penis] is *Gou Jing* (Dog Essence). [Dogs] grow in plains and swamps.

Lu Rong **(Cornu Parvum Cervi)**[331] is sweet and warm. It mainly treats leaking of malign blood and cold and heat fright epilepsy. It boosts the qi, fortifies the will, promotes the growth of the teeth, and prevents senility.

---

[328] The identity of this medicinal is not clear.

[329] This is a general term for various categories of women's disease. In premodern times, sometimes any gynecological disease was spoken of as *dai xia bing* (literally, below the belt disease).

[330] Dog Gall may be used to treat nosebleed, scarring sores, malign sores, deep-source nasal congestion, nasal polyps, blood stasis caused by falls and knocks, and incised wounds. To treat eye diseases, one may administer it with wine.

[331] This medicinal supplements the essence and boosts the qi, fortifies the sinews and strengthens the bones. It is a good medicinal for pain in the lumbus and knees, dizziness, blurred vision, flooding, seminal emission, and all kinds of vacuity taxation. In his explanation of this passage, Ye Gui said:

> When the liver cannot store the blood, the spleen will be unable to govern the blood. In consequence, leaking of malign blood arises. Velvet Deerhorn is warm of qi and, as such, is able to reach the liver. Because it is sweet in flavor, it can support the spleen. For that reason, it is a remedy for this condition. Cold and heat fright epilepsy is fright epilepsy complicated by cold and heat. When there is liver blood vacuity, the liver qi will be hyperactive and bring turbidity fire upward. Because Velvet Deerhorn nourishes the blood and abducts fire, it checks fright epilepsy and [accompanying] cold and heat...

121

The horn [Cornu Cervi][332] mainly treats malign sores, welling abscesses, and swellings and expels evil malign qi and lodged blood in the genitals.

Fu Yi (**Vesperugo Noctula**)[333] is salty and balanced. It mainly treats heavy eyes, brightens the eyes, and furnishes them with spirit light at night. Protracted taking may make one happy, elevated, and worry-free. Its other name is *Bian Fu* (Flat Wing). It grows in the rivers and valleys of Tai Shan.

Wei Pi (**Pellis Erinacei**)[334] is bitter and balanced. It mainly treats the five [kinds of] hemorrhoids, genital erosion, red and white blood precipitation [*i.e.*, dysentery], incessant hemafecia of the five colors, and genital swelling and pain radiating to the upper and lower back. One should kill [the hedgehog] by boiling it in wine [in order to remove its skin]. It grows in rivers and valleys.

Shi Long Zi (**Eumeces Seu Sphenomorphus**) is salty and cold. It mainly treats the five dribbling urinary stoppages and evil bound qi, breaks stone strangury, precipitates the blood, and disinhibits urination and the water

---

[332] Deerhorn (*Lu Jiao*) has nearly the same actions as Velvet Deerhorn (*Lu Rong*), and, since it is much cheaper, it is often substituted for the latter. When administered unprocessed, it treats malaria in children and dream intercourse with ghosts. After being ground with vinegar, it is able to disperse swelling toxins and bedsores. When powdered, it treats fractures and injured sinews. After being cooked, it boosts the essence, supplements the kidneys, and quickens the blood. Therefore, it is used to treat frequent urination, lower burner wasting thirst, and pain in the lumbar spine. Mixed with pig fat, it can heal all sorts of cinnabar toxins. After being ground in water, it disperses swelling toxins.

[333] Bat is said to be a remedy for any category of strangury besides what is explained in the text. In ancient times, bats were worshipped as a divine medicinal and were described as having some miraculous effects. Some Daoists took bat eyes and gall in the hope of acquiring special physical abilities, particularly good eyesight and night vision.

[334] Hedgehog Pelt has the actions of cooling the blood, opening the stomach, and astringing. In addition to those indications mentioned in the text, it is a wonderful remedy for any kind of seminal emission, including dream emission, vacuity or repletion emission, and seminal efflux.

passageways. Its other name is *Xi Yi* (Rare Snake). It grows in rivers and valleys.

Sang Piao Xiao (**Ootheca Mantidis**)[335] is salty and balanced. It mainly treats damaged center, mounting conglomeration, and impotence. It boosts the essence, makes pregnancy possible, [cures] blood block and lumbago in females, frees the five stranguries, and disinhibits urination and the water passageways. It grows on mulberry twigs. It should be steamed after being collected [for use]. Its other name is *Shi You* (Eroding Wart).

Zhai Chan (**Cicada**)[336] is salty and cold. It mainly treats fright epilepsy and night crying in children, madness, and cold and heat. It grows in poplar and willow trees.

Bai Jiang Can (**Bombyx Batryticatus**)[337] is salty. It mainly treats fright epilepsy and night crying in children, removes three [kinds of] worms, and eliminates black patches on the face, thus making the facial complexion attractive, and genital sores in males. It grows in plains and swamps.

Mu Mang (**Tabanus Trigonus**) is bitter and balanced. It mainly treats sore, red eyes, injured canthi, tearing, blood stasis, blood block, cold and heat,

---

[335] Mantis Egg-case is able to boost the essence and secure the kidneys. Nowadays, it is mainly used for children's bed-wetting, seminal emission, and frequent urination. For these purposes, it can be used singly. A famous formula with Mantis Egg-case as the sovereign ingredient is called *Sang Piao Xiao San* (Mantis Egg-Case Powder). It is capable of quieting the heart and spirit, improving memory, and astringing frequent voidings of urine.

[336] Cicada per se is seldom used. Instead, *Chan Tui* (Periostracum Cicadae), which has the same actions, is prescribed to treat intense fevers, eye screen, and slow progression or non-eruption of papules in addition to what is discussed in the text above.

[337] *Bai Jiang Can* refers to Silkworm killed by fungus. It is now considered acrid and salty in flavor and slightly warm of qi. It is able to expel wind and transform phlegm, dissipate binding and move the channels. It is often used in wind stroke with loss of voice, head wind, toothache, throat impediment, cinnabar toxins, itchy sores, fistulas, flooding and vaginal discharge, fright epilepsy, *gan*, and difficult lactation. In addition, it is able to eliminate scars.

aching, and infertility. Its other name is *Hun Chang* (Constant Soul). It grows in rivers and swamps.

Fei Mang (**Tabanus Bovinus**) is bitter and slightly cold. It mainly expels blood stasis, breaks precipitating blood [sic],[338] accumulations, hard glomus, concretions and conglomerations with cold and heat, and frees and disinhibits the blood vessels and the nine orifices. It grows in rivers and valleys.

Fei Lian (**Stylopyga Conucina**) is salty. It mainly treats blood stasis, concretions and hardness with cold and heat, breaks gatherings and accumulations, and [cures] throat impediment and internal cold infertility. It grows in rivers and swamps.

Qi Cao (**Holotrichia Diomphalia**) is salty and slightly warm. It mainly treats malign blood, blood stasis, and impediment qi, breaks decayed blood in the rib-side giving rise to fullness and pain, and [cures] menstrual block, outcrop, green-blue screen, and white membrane in the eye. Its other name is *Fen Qi* (Mound Worm). It grows in plains and swamps.

Kuo Yu (**Limax**) is salty and cold. It mainly treats bandit wind [giving rise to] deviated eyes and mouth, cramps, prolapse of the rectum, fright epilepsy, and hypertonicity. Its other name is *Ling Li* (Mound Woodworm). It grows in pools and swamps.

Hai Ge (**Concha Cyclinae Sinensis**)[339] is bitter and balanced. It mainly treats cough and counterflow qi ascent, panting, vexatious fullness, chest pain, and cold and heat. Its other name is *Kui Ge* (Bulky Shell). It grows in

---

[338] The text seems to be garbled here. This line probably should read, "precipitating the blood and breaking hard gatherings..."

[339] The current name of this medicinal is (*Hai*) *Ge Fen*, Clam Shell Powder. It has the same actions as *Mu Li* (Concha Ostreae). It treats chest pain, vexatious fullness, water qi puffy swelling, cough and panting, impotence, flooding and vaginal discharge, goiters and tumors, and hemorrhoids. In addition, it quenches thirst and resolves hangover. *Wen Ge* is a particular species of *Hai Ge*. It may be Cythica Meretrix, Psammobia, or Sunetta Excavata. It seems to have a wider range of actions than *Hai Ge*. For example, sores are also included under its indications.

pools and swamps. *Wen Ge* (Concha Cythircae Meretricis) mainly treats malign sores and the five [kinds of] eroding hemorrhoids.

Gui Jia **(Plastrum Testudinis)**[340] is salty and balanced. It mainly treats red and white leaking, breaks concretions and conglomerations, and [cures] malaria, the five hemorrhoids, genital erosion, damp impediment, heaviness and weakness of the limbs, and non-closure of the fontanel in children. Protracted taking may make the body light and free from hunger. Its other name is *Shen Wu* (God House). It is produced in pools and swamps.

Bie Jia **(Carapax Amydae Sinensis)**[341] is salty and balanced. It mainly treats heart and abdominal concretions and conglomerations and hard

---

[340] The current name of this medicinal is *Gui Ban*. It supplements the heart and boosts the kidneys, enriches yin and clears heat. Besides those illnesses listed in the text, it treats blood vacuity, taxation fever, steaming bones, pain in the lumbus and legs, enduring cough, enduring malaria, and concretions and conglomerations. It is a wonderful medicinal for yin vacuity and blood debility. Chen Nian-zhu said:

> All people say that it greatly supplements true water and, therefore, ranks first in divinely yin-enriching medicinals. In my opinion, this is [only] a view. Generally speaking, animals with shells are all attributed to yin and, as such, are able to eliminate heat. Those growing in water are all capable of disinhibiting dampness. Shells [also] correspond to metal and, therefore, are able to whittle away hardness.

To enrich yin, Tortoise Plastron can be administered for a long time, usually in the form of gelatin. To treat steaming bones, it is prescribed together with Phellodendron and Anemarrhena. To supplement both yin and yang, one may use it in combination with Deerhorn. If it is used together with Biota Leaves and Cyperus, it dissipates depression and binding. In case of nonmovement of the coccyx in childbirth, one may administer it together with carbonized Human Hair, Dang Gui, and Ligusticum Wallichium.

[341] Turtle Shell has nearly the same actions as Tortoise Plastron but is more effective. It supplements yin, dissipates binding, and clears heat. Turtle Shell is found in a great many proven formulas. As a group, internally, these formulas treat taxation damage, malaria, lumbago, difficult delivery, concretions and conglomerations, and intestinal abscess, and, externally, they cure hemorrhoids, prolapse of the rectum, and genital swelling and sores.

accumulations with cold and heat. It removes glomus, polyps, genital erosion, hemorrhoids, and malign flesh. It is produced in pools and swamps.

Tuo Yu Jia (**Squama Alligator Sinensis**) is acrid and slightly warm. It mainly treats heart and abdominal concretions and conglomerations, deep-lying hard accumulations and gatherings, cold and heat, flooding and blood precipitation of the five colors in females, contracting pain between the lower abdomen and genitals, sores, scabs, and dead muscles. It is produced in pools and swamps.

Wu Zei Yu Gu (**Os Sepiae Seu Sepiellae**)[342] is salty and slightly warm. It mainly cures women's leaking, red and white menses, blood block, genital erosion, swelling and pain, cold and heat, concretions and conglomerations, and infertility. It is produced in pools and swamps.

Xie (**Eriocheir Sinensis**)[343] is salty and cold. It mainly treats evil qi in the chest, bound heat pain, deviated mouth and eyes, and swollen face. It overcomes lacquer [toxins]. When burnt, it may attract mice. It grows in pools and swamps.

---

[342] The current name of this medicinal is *Hai Piao Xiao*. Squid Bone frees the flow of the blood vessels, expels cold dampness, and enriches desiccated blood. Besides the indications discussed in the text, it is also effective for purulent ear and eye diseases such as eye screen.

[343] This refers to fresh water crabs. According to the text, the whole of the crab is used as a medicinal. In present-day clinical practice, its flesh, shell, eggs, and chelae are all prescribed as separate medicinals. However, the only one of these frequently used is Crab Chelae. This is often administered to induce abortion or hasten delivery. Sometimes Crab Eggs are applied to heal lacquer sores.

Xia Ma **(Bufo Bufo)**[344] is acrid and cold. It mainly treats evil qi, breaks concretions, hardness, and the blood and [heals] welling abscesses and swellings and genital sores. Taking it may prevent febrile diseases. It grows in pools and swamps.

---

[344] The current name of this medicinal is *Chan Chu*. One should note that in modern Chinese, *Xia Ma* is frog. Nowadays whole toad is seldom prescribed. Instead, *Chan Su* (Secretio Bufonis) is often used. *Chan Su* is efficacious for various sores, including clove sores, and for children's *gan* in general and brain *gan* in particular. The symptoms of brain *gan* include head sores, fever, loss of hair, dry nose, parched lips, and lusterless eyes.

Animals: Inferior Class

Liu Chu Mao Ti Jia (Hair & Hooves of the Six Species of Domesticated Animals)[345] are salty and balanced. It mainly treats demonic influx, *gu* toxins, cold and heat, fright epilepsy, withdrawal, tetany, and manic running about. The hair of the camel is particularly good [for the above diseases].

Lei Shu (Trogopterus Seu Pteromys)[346] mainly induces abortion and makes delivery smooth.

Mi Zhi (Adeps Elaphuri Davidiani)[347] is acrid and warm. It mainly treats welling abscesses and swellings, malign sores, dead muscles, cold wind

---

[345] It seems odd to the translator that the author discusses the six species of domesticated animals in a single lump since some parts of them are discussed in the previous and following passages. The six categories of animals referred to are the horse, cow, sheep, pig, dog, and chicken. However, it seems that other domesticated animals are also referred to here, for example, the camel. Unlike this classic, later materia medica usually treat the six categories of animals in terms of their parts under separate headings. Since this work deals with them indiscriminately, we cannot tell exactly what is the medical effect of a particular part of a particular animal. In addition, we cannot tell whether the claws and feathers of the chicken should be included under "hooves and hair."

[346] Because this passage is so short, lacking even the origin of the medicinal, it is probable that it has been corrupted from the original. In an annotation on this passage, Tao Hong-jing said, "Make the birthing woman hold the pelt of the flying squirrel and she will have smooth delivery."

[347] Various parts of the David's Deer (or *Mi Lu*), such as the horn and bone, were more commonly used as separate medicinals than the flesh. In modern clinical practice, however, none of these are often prescribed because this species of deer has long been near to extinction.

damp impediment, hypertonicity and loss of use of the limbs, head wind, and swelling qi. It frees the interstices. Its other name is *Gong Zhi* (Palace Fat). It is produced in mountains and valleys.

Tun Nuan (Testes Suis)[348] is sweet and warm. It mainly treats fright epilepsy, madness, demonic influx, and *gu* toxins. It eliminates cold and heat, running piglet, the five dribbling urinary blocks, evil qi, and [muscle] contracture. The hind shoes [*i.e.*, the outer part of the foot] mainly treats the five [kinds of] hemorrhoids, hidden heat in the intestines, intestinal abscess, and internal erosion. [Pig Testes] are also called *Tun Dian* (Pig Summit).

Yan Shi (Excrementum Hirundi Rusticae Gutturalis) is acrid and balanced. It mainly treats *gu* toxins and demonic influx, expels ill matters and evil qi, breaks the five dribbling urinary blocks, and disinhibits urination. It is produced in high mountains and low valleys.[349]

Tian Shu Shi (Excrementum Verpertilionis Murini)[350] is acrid and cold. It mainly treats welling abscesses and swelling of the face and eyes, continual pain in the skin, and blood qi in the abdomen. It breaks accumulations and gatherings with cold and heat and eliminates fright epilepsy. Its other name is *Shu Gu* (Mouse Droppings). Yet another name is *Shi Gan* (Stone Liver). It is produced in the mountains and valleys of He Pu.[351]

---

[348] There is no consensus in China about the identity of this medicinal. Li Shi-zhen thought it to be the testicles of the young pig, while another view says it is none other than the young pig itself.

[349] Swallows usually build their nests in houses, not in mountains and valleys.

[350] The current name of this medicinal is *Ye Ming Sha*. Its actions include quickening the blood and brightening the eyes. In modern prescriptions, it is mainly used to treat eye diseases, like night blindness, screen, and obstruction. Nevertheless, the other indications listed in the text are valid.

[351] This is a place in present-day Guangdong Province.

Lu Feng Fang (**Nidus Vespae**)[352] is bitter and balanced. It mainly treats fright epilepsy, tuggings and slackenings, cold and heat, evil qi, madness, ghost essence, *gu* toxins, and intestinal hemorrhoids.[353] It is better if it is baked [for use]. Its other name is *Feng Chang* (Wasp Hovel). It is produced in mountains and valleys.

Hua Ji (**Mecopoda Elongata**) is bitter and balanced. It mainly treats heart and abdominal evil qi and impotence, boosts the essence, fortifies the will, makes pregnancy possible, and renders the facial complexion attractive. It supplements the center and makes the body light. It grows in rivers and valleys.

Zhe Chong (**Eupolyphaga Seu Opisthoplatia**)[354] is salty and cold. It mainly treats heart and abdominal continual cold and heat, blood accumulation, and concretions and conglomerations. It breaks hardness and precipitates blood block. The offspring is usually good.[355] Its other name is *Di Bie* (Underground Tortoise). It grows in rivers and valleys.

Shui Zhi (**Hirudo Seu Whitmania**) is salty and balanced. It mainly expels malign blood, blood stasis, and menstrual block, breaks blood

---

[352] Administration of this medicinal together with Snake Slough and carbonized Human Hair can heal deep-to-the-bone flat abscesses (*fu gu ju*). To treat fistulas, one may mix it with pig fat and apply. After it is boiled in lime water, it can cure jealous milk. This is an illness due to too copious milk or retained milk in the breast. It is characterized by swelling and pain in the breast with tangible nodes. In addition, it may treat double tongue, toothache, and impotence. Nowadays, it is mainly used for scrofulas. It can also make bathwater to treat sudden epilepsy in children. Bathe the ill child in it, and the child will be relieved of the disease immediately.

[353] *I.e.*, anal swelling and suppuration

[354] Wingless Cockroach is particularly good at breaking lodged blood and gatherings and accumulations, dispersing swelling, and promoting lactation. It also treats swollen tongue. In terms of the source of this insect, it actually grows everywhere.

[355] The Chinese is *sheng zi da liang*. The meaning of this phrase is rather confusing. Its literal translation is, "[It] gives birth to a greatly good child."

conglomerations, accumulations and gatherings, [treats] infertility [due to blood stasis], and disinhibits the water passageways. It grows in lakes and swamps.

Shi Can (**Phryganea Japonica**) is sour. It is nontoxic. It mainly treats the five dribbling urinary blocks, breaks stone strangury, and induces abortion. Its flesh[356] resolves bound qi, disinhibits the water passageways, and eliminates heat. Its other name is *Sha Shi* (Sand Louse). It grows in pools and swamps.

She Tui (**Exuviae Serpentis**)[357] is salty and balanced. It mainly treats the 120 categories of fright epilepsy, and tuggings and slackenings in children, and madness, cold and heat, intestinal hemorrhoids, worm toxins, and snake epilepsy. It is better if it is baked [for use]. Its other name is *Long Zi Yi* (Robe of the Baby Dragon). Yet another name is *She Fu* (Snake Talisman). It is also called *Long Zi Dan Yi* (Shirt of the Baby Dragon) and *Gong Pi* (Bow Cover). It is produced in rivers and valleys.

Wu Gong (**Scolopendra Subspinipes**)[358] is acrid and warm. It mainly treats demonic influx, *gu* toxins, and snake, worm, and fish toxins. It kills demonic matters, [treats] old essence and warm malaria, and removes the three [kinds of] worms. It grows in rivers and valleys.

Ma Lu (**Prospirobolus Johannsis**) is acrid and warm. It mainly treats large-sized hard concretions, breaks accumulations and gatherings, and

---

[356] Because this insect is very small, it must be very difficult to separate its flesh. Hence, the translator suspects that there is something wrong with this passage.

[357] Snake Slough effuses the exterior, expels wind, resolves toxins, and removes eye screen. It is used to treat fright epilepsy, wind malaria, throat impediment, double tongue, lockjaw, sores, and hemorrhoids. It is often burned and powdered for use to treat external troubles like malign sores and throat impediment.

[358] Centipede is a good medicinal for expelling wind, killing parasites, and inducing abortion. To treat cinnabar toxin tumor, one may mix powdered Centipede with Alum, Omphalia, and Radix Stemonae (*Bai Bu*). To treat clenched jaw in newborns, administer stir-fried Centipede powder mixed with pig milk.

[heals] polyps, malign sores, and white bald scalp sores. Its other name is *Bai Zu* (Hundred Feet). It grows in rivers and valleys.

Yi Weng (**Eumenes Pomifomis**) is acrid and balanced. It mainly treats enduring deafness, cough and counterflow, and toxic qi. It helps extract thorns [in the flesh] and promotes sweating. It grows in rivers and valleys.

Que Weng (**Cocoon of Monema Flavescens**) is sweet and balanced. It mainly treats fright epilepsy in children, cold and heat bound qi, *gu* toxins, and demonic influx. Its other name is *Zao She* (Agitating House).

Bi Zi (**Rana Nigromaculata**)[359] is sweet and warm. It mainly treats evil qi in the abdomen and it removes the three [kinds of] worms, snakebite [toxins], *gu* toxins, demonic influx, and hidden corpse.

Shu Fu (**Armadillidium Vulgare**) is sour and warm. It mainly treats qi dribbling urinary block, menstrual block and blood conglomeration in females, epilepsy, tetany, and cold and heat. It disinhibits the water passageways. Its other name is *Pan Fu* (Crooked Woman). Yet another name is *Yi Wei* (Woman's Dignity). It grows in plains and valleys.

Ying Huo (**Luciola Vitticollis**) is acrid and slightly warm. It mainly brightens the eyes, [heals] fire sores and burns in children, and [treats] heat qi, *gu* toxins, and demonic influx. It [also] frees the spirit essence.[360] Its other name is *Ye Guang* (Night Light). It grows in pools and swamps.

Yi Yu (**Lepisma Saccharina**) is salty and warm. It is nontoxic, mainly treating mounting conglomeration in females, inhibited urination, and wind stroke with rigidity of the neck in children. [To treat the above,] it

---

[359] The identity of this medicinal is uncertain. There are various speculations about it. One of them even suggests that it is *Fei Zi* (Semen Torreyae), saying it is not an animal or part of an animal at all. Some specialists believe it to be *Xia Ma* (Bufo Bufo).

[360] Spirit essence here means the eyes. Therefore, this sentence implies that the Firefly may make the eyes bright.

should be rubbed [over the affected area]. Its other name is *Bai Yu* (White Fish). It grows in plains and swamps.

Bai Jing Qiu Yin (**Lumbricus**)[361] is salty and cold. It mainly treats snake [toxins] and conglomerations. It removes the three [kinds of] worms, hidden corpse, demonic influx, and *gu* toxins, and it kills long worms [*i.e.*, tapeworms]. It transforms back into water by itself.[362] It grows in the earth in the plains.

Lou Gu (**Gryllotalpa Africana**)[363] is salty and cold. It mainly treats difficult delivery, helps extract thorns in the flesh, opens welling abscesses and swellings, precipitates [bones] stuck in the throat and dysphagia, resolves toxins, and eliminates malign sores. Those that are caught crawling out are better. Its other name is *Hui Gu* (Gentle Ant). Yet another name is *Tian Lou* (Celestial Chirping Insect). It is also called *Gu* (Digger). It grows in plains and swamps.

Qiang Lang (**Geotrupes Laesistriatus**) is salty and cold. It mainly treats fright epilepsy, tuggings and slackenings, abdominal distention, cold and heat in children, and withdrawal and mania in adults. It is better if baked

---

[361] The current name of this medicinal is *Di Long* (Earth Dragon). In the name in this text, the characters *Bai Jing* mean white neck. This suggests that one should use old Earthworms as medicinals. Besides the indications listed in the text, Earthworms can treat warm disease with intense fever and delirium, wind stroke, epilepsy, throat impediment, and febrile disease.

[362] This implies that if the Earthworm is salted and exposed to the sun, it will immediately give off copious fluids.

[363] Tao Hong-jing said in his annotation to this passage:

Its upper part is rather astringing and, therefore, mainly stops urination and defecation [*i.e.*, enuresis and diarrhea]. Its lower part is rather lubricating and, therefore, mainly precipitates the urine and stools. To extract thorns in the flesh, its brain is usually used.

In the *Sheng Hui Fang* (*Sagelike Prescriptions from the Great Grace Era*) compiled by Chen Zhao-yu and Wang Huai-yin in 992 CE, this medicinal is said to be able to cure all categories of water disease, including strangury.

[for use]. Its other name is *Jie Qiang* (Strong Feet). It grows in pools and swamps.

Ban Mao (Mylabris) is acrid and cold. It mainly treats cold and heat, demonic influx, *gu* toxins, mouse fistulas, malign sores, flat abscesses and erosion, and dead muscles. [In addition,] it breaks stone dribbling urinary block.[364] Its other name is *Long Wei* (Dragon Tail). It grows in rivers and valleys.

Di Dan (Meloe Coartatus) is acrid and cold. It mainly treats demonic influx, cold and heat, mouse fistulas, malign sores, and dead muscles. It breaks concretions and conglomerations and induces abortion. Its other name is *Yuan Qing* (Original Green-blue). It grows in rivers and valleys.

Ma Dao (Mactra Quandrangularis) is acrid and slightly cold. It is toxic, mainly treating leaking and red and white [vaginal discharge] and cold and heat. It breaks stone strangury and kills fowl, beasts, and bandit mice. It grows in pools and swamps.

Bei Zi (Cypraea Macula)[365] is salty and balanced. It mainly treats eye screen, demonic influx, *gu* toxins, and abdominal pain. It precipitates the blood, [heals] the five dribbling urinary blocks, and disinhibits the water passageways. It is better if burnt [for use]. It grows in pools and swamps.

---

[364] This may refer to stone strangury or urinary lithiasis in modern terms.

[365] This is a species of shellfish which is very small. However, it may include several different subspecies, like Cypraea Moneta, Cypraea Zicraea, and Cypraea Asellus.

Fruits and Vegetables: Superior Class

Pu Tao (**Fructus Viticis Viniferae**) is sweet and balanced. It mainly treats sinew and bone damp impediment, boosts the qi, doubles the [physical] force, fortifies the will, makes one fat, strong, and able to endure hunger and wind cold. Protracted taking may make the body light and never senile and prolong life. It can be made into wine. It grows in mountains and valleys.

Peng Lei (**Fructus Rubi Chingii**) is sour and balanced. It mainly quiets the five viscera, boosts the essence qi, promotes the growth of and strengthens yin, fortifies the will, doubles [physical] force, and makes pregnancy possible. Protracted taking may make the body light and prevent senility. Its other name is *Fu Pen* (Upside-down Basin). It grows in plains and swamps.

Da Zao (**Fructus Zizyphi Jujubae**)[366] is sweet and balanced. It mainly

---

[366] Among the many actions of this medicinal recorded in the Chinese materia medica literature to date, the most important ones are to nourish the spleen and boost the lungs and stomach. The spleen and lungs govern all the qi throughout the body, while the spleen also governs all the blood. Since this medicinal is able to harmonize the blood and qi, it is good for almost any condition. Generally speaking, Red Dates, which are sweet, are relaxing and moderating. Although they are able to disinhibit the nine orifices, they work temperately and slowly. When helped by the acrid of Ginger, their relaxing effect is modified. Ginger rules the defensive, while Red Dates govern the constructive. Thus the combination of the two harmonizes the constructive and defensive. Hence, we can find these two medicinals side by side in many formulas. When discussing the effects of Red Dates, Zou Shu said:

When cold evils strike a person, the central qi may be too insufficient to expel them. This is because there is shortage of qi. When heat evils strike

(continued...)

treats heart and abdominal evil qi, quiets the center and nourishes the spleen, assists the 12 channels, levels the stomach qi, frees the nine orifices, supplements shortage of qi, shortage of fluids, and insufficiency of the body, [eliminates] great fright and heaviness of the limbs, and harmonizes hundreds of medicinals. Protracted taking may make the body light and lengthen life. Together with Herba Ephedrae, its leaf [Folium Zizyphi Jujubae] is able to promote sweating. It grows in plains and swamps.

Ou Shi Jing (**Semen Et Nodus Rhizomatis Nelumbinis Nuciferae**)[367] is

---

[366](...continued)

a person, the central qi may [also] be too insufficient to expel them. This is because there is shortage of fluids. When the pulse is bound and regularly interrupted and there is stirring palpitations of the heart, this is because of insufficiency of the qi of the 12 channels. When fire counterflows with qi ascent, there will arise inhibited throat, insufficiency of fluids, unbalanced stomach qi, and disharmony of the nine orifices. Thanks to their magnificent action of quieting the center, [Red Dates] are able to put an end to chaotic qi. Then great fright will be eliminated. Thanks to their magnificent action of pushing and moving the 12 channels, the channel qi will be set in motion without any more stagnation. Then heaviness of the limbs will be eliminated. Red Dates are allowed into a dissipating prescription in order to quiet the center, nourish the spleen, and level the stomach. In supplementing prescriptions, they may also be found for the purpose of assisting the channel qi to eliminate evil qi. This is what is meant by their ability to harmonize hundreds of medicinals.

[367] The current name of Semen Nelumbinis Nuciferae is *Lian Zi* or *Lian Rou* and that of Nodus Rhizomatis Nelumbinis Nuciferae is *Ou* or *Ou Jie*. In modern prescriptions, they have different actions. Lotus Seed fortifies the spleen and the stomach and quiets the heart and spirit. It is used to treat noninteraction between the heart and kidneys, enduring dysentery, seminal emission, turbid urine, flooding, vaginal discharge, and other blood troubles. Ye Gui explained:

Being sweet in flavor and balanced of qi, it supplements the center. Because it is fragrant and hence able to clear the heart, it nurtures the spirit. Sweetness and balanced [qi] may boost the spleen and lungs. Therefore, it boosts the physical force. The heart is the governor of the 12 organs. So long as the governor is quiet, the 12 organs are quiet. It follows that none of the hundreds of diseases can persist.

(continued...)

138

sweet and balanced. It mainly supplements the center and nourishes the spirit, boosts the qi and [physical] force, and eliminates hundreds of diseases. Protracted taking may make the body light, slow aging, make one free from hunger, and prolong life. Its other name is *Shui Zhi* (Water Ganomdera). It grows in pools and swamps.

Ji Tou (**Semen Euryalis Ferocis**)[368] is sweet and balanced. It mainly treats damp impediment and pain in the lumbar spine and knees, supplements the center, eliminates hundreds of diseases, boosts the essence qi, fortifies the will, and sharpens the ears and eyes. Protracted taking may make the body light and free from hunger, and slow aging to make one an immortal.

Gan Gua Zi (**Semen Benincasae Hispidae**)[369] is sweet and balanced. It mainly renders the facial complexion shiny and attractive, boosts the qi, and makes one free from hunger. Protracted taking may make the body

---

[367](...continued)
Lotus Root cools the blood and dissipates stasis, eliminates vexation and quenches thirst. It is often used to staunch blood ejection and nosebleed and cure strangury and dysentery. In fact, it is a remedy for any troubles related to blood.

[368] The current name of this medicinal is *Qian Shi*. It secures the kidneys and boosts the essence, supplements the spleen and eliminates dampness. It is a good medicinal for original yang vacuity and cold, diarrhea, vaginal discharge, turbid urine, urinary incontinence, dream seminal emission, seminal efflux, and cold pain in the lumbus and knees. When combined with Cuscuta Seed, it solidifies the stools. Together with Rehmannia, it cures all sorts of bleeding. *Shui Lu Er Xian Gao* (Water & Land Immortals Paste), composed of Cherokee Rose Fruit besides Euryales Seed, is an effective formula for kidney cold, seminal emission, and vaginal discharge.

[369] The Chinese word *gan* means sweet. Therefore, this medicinal should be Melon Seed (Semen Curcumeris). However, some distinguished scholars, such as Su Jing who lived in the Tang dynasty, have thought otherwise, identifying it as *Dong Gua Zi* (Semen Benincasae Hispidae). *Dong Gua Zi* is able to eliminate vexation, fullness, melancholy, the five taxations and seven damages, and enduring sores. In addition, it is also able to brighten the eyes and moisten the skin to render the facial complexion attractive. *Gua Di*, although standing side by side with Semen Benincasae Hispidae in the same passage, is undoubtedly Pediculus Curcumeris. Melon Stalk now is mainly used as an emetic to treat wind phlegm, abiding food, etc.

139

light and slow aging. *Gua Di* (Pediculus Curcumeris) is bitter and cold. It mainly treats great water [giving rise to] puffy swelling of the trunk, face, and limbs. It precipitates water, kills *gu* toxins, and [suppresses] cough and counterflow qi ascent. It provokes ejection to precipitate diseases located in the chest and abdomen due to nondispersion of various fruits. Its other name is *Tu Zhi* (Earth Ganoderma). These grow in plains and swamps.

Dong Kui Zi (**Semen Abutilonis Seu Malvae**) is sweet and cold. It mainly treats cold and heat, languor and emaciation due to the five viscera and six bowels, breaks the five stranguries, and disinhibits urination. Protracted taking may fortify the bones, promote the growth of the muscles and flesh, make the body light, and prolong life.

Xian Shi (**Semen Amaranthi**)[370] is sweet and cold. It mainly treats clear-eye blindness, brightens the eyes, eliminates evils, disinhibits urination and defecation, and relieves cold and heat. Protracted taking may boost the qi and [physical] force and make one free from hunger and the body light. Its other name is *Ma Xian* (Horse Wild Herb). It grows in plains and swamps.

Ku Cai (**Herba Sonchi Oleracei**) is bitter and cold. It mainly treats evils in the five viscera, aversion to grain, and stomach impediment. Protracted taking may quiet the heart, boost the qi, sharpen the senses, lessen sleep, make the body light, and slow aging. Its other name is *Tu Cao* (Rampant Weed). Yet another name is *Xuan* (Choice). It grows in rivers and valleys.

---

[370] This plant should not be confused with *Ma Chi Xian* (Portulaca Oleracea) although their Chinese names sound similar.

Fruits and Vegetables: Middle Class

Ying Tao (**Fructus Pruni Pseudocerasi**) is sweet and balanced. It is nontoxic, mainly regulating the center and boosting the spleen qi. It may render the facial complexion attractive and glorify one's will.[371]

Mei Shi (**Fructus Pruni Mume**)[372] is sour and balanced. It mainly precipitates the qi, eliminates heat and vexatious fullness, quiets the heart, [relieves] pain in the limbs, hemilateral withering with insensitivity, and dead muscles, and removes green-blue and black moles and malign diseases. It grows in rivers and valleys.

Liao Shi (**Fructus Polygoni Hydropiperis**) is acrid and warm. It mainly brightens the eyes, warms the center, helps endure wind cold, precipitates water qi to treat puffy swelling of the face and eyes, and [heals] welling abscesses and sores. *Ma Liao* (Herba Polygoni Blumei) eliminates leeches from the intestines and makes the body light. [They] grow in rivers and valleys.

---

[371] If rendered connotatively, the word *zhi* (will) means intention, desire, or aspiration. Among fruits, Cherry ripens earliest in the year. Therefore, in olden times, it was regarded the best of the fruits as a sacrifice to the gods, *i.e.*, a first fruit. This may be what is implied in this phrase.

[372] The current name is *Wu Mei*. It astringes the lung qi and intestines, generates fluids and quenches thirst, resolves hangover and kills parasites. In his *Ri Hua Zi*, Da Ming of the Tang dynasty, said, "It treats steaming bones and eliminates vexation and oppression, hemilateral withering, and insensitivity of the skin." To treat blood dysentery, it should be combined with Coptis and Terra Flava Usta. If it is prescribed together with Ginger and *Shen Qu* (Massa Medica Fermentata), it treats intermittent dysentery. After being boiled, it is able to cure intense heart and abdominal distention and pain. There is a formula called *Wu Mei Wan* (Mume Pills) composed of nothing but Mume. It is good for roundworm reversal with cold limbs and great abdominal pain.

Cong Shi **(Semen Allii Fistulosi)**[373] is acrid and warm. It mainly brightens the eyes and supplements center insufficiency. The stalk [Bulbus Allii Fistulosi], which can be made into soup, mainly treats cold damage cold and heat. It promotes sweating and [cures] wind stroke swollen face and eyes. *Xie Bai* (Bulbus Allii)[374] is acrid and mainly treats incised wounds and suppurating wounds. It may make the body light and [the taker] free from hunger and slow aging. [They] grow in plains and swamps.

Shui Su **(Herba Stachydis Baicalensis)**[375] is acrid and slightly warm. It mainly precipitates the qi, kills [*i.e.*, disperses] grain, gets rid of bad breath, eliminates toxins, and keeps off malign qi.[376] Protracted taking may enable one to communicate with the spirit light, make the body light, and slow aging. It grows in pools and swamps.

---

[373] In modern prescriptions, Chinese Scallion Seed is rarely if ever used as a medicinal, but *Cong Bai* (Bulbus Allii Fistulosi) is in wide use. When discussing the actions of *Cong Bai*, Tao Hong-jing said:

> It mainly treats bone and flesh pain in cold damage and throat impediment with block. It quiets the fetus, brightens the eyes, eliminates evil qi in the liver, quiets the center, disinhibits the five viscera, boosts the eye essence, and resolves the toxins of hundreds of medicinals.

[374] *Xie* (Allium Macrostemum) is acrid and bitter in flavor and warm of qi. In most cases, *Xie Bai* (Bulbus Allii) is used. *Xie* treats chest impediment pain, diarrhea, dysentery, panting, scalds, and sores. Besides, it is often used to treat bones stuck in the throat and the swallowing of foreign substances.

[375] In addition to the indications discussed in the text, this medicinal also treats various blood troubles, such as blood ejection, hemafecia, and flooding and leaking.

[376] Here, malign qi means bad breath.

Xing He (**Semen Pruni Armeniacae**)[377] is sweet and warm. It mainly treats cough and counterflow qi ascent, thunderous rumbling [of the intestines], and throat impediment. It precipitates the qi, promotes lactation, and [heals] incised wounds, cold heart, and running piglet. It grows in rivers and valleys.

---

[377] The current name of this medicinal is *Xing Ren*. Apricot Seeds are a widely used medicinal. They drain the lungs and resolve the muscles, eliminate wind and dissipate cold, downbear the qi and move phlegm, disperse food accumulation and free the qi in constipation due to the large intestine. Because they are able to eliminate wind heat in the lungs, they are often used to treat cold damage with rigidity and pain in the head and neck, panting and absence of sweat. For this purpose, they are prescribed together with Ephedrae, Cinnamon Twigs, and Licorice. To suppress panting, level qi, and promote sweating, one may administer them together with Ephedra. For chest binding with pain, hardness, and distention of the upper abdomen, one may use them together with Mirabilitum and Honey. Moreover, they are frequently applied externally. Smashed, they heal swollen face and suppuration of the nose.

Fruits and Vegetables: Inferior Class

Tao He (**Semen Pruni Persicae**)[378] is bitter and balanced. It mainly treats blood stasis, blood block, conglomerations, and evil qi. It kills small worms. *Tao Hua* (Flos Pruni Persicae) kills malign demonic influx and gives one a good facial complexion. *Tao Xiao* (old Fructus Pruni Persicae)[379] is slightly warm. It kills hundreds of ghosts and spiritual matters. *Tao Mao* (Peach Fuzz) mainly precipitates blood conglomerations, accumulations and gatherings with cold and heat and [cures] infertility. *Tao Du* (Peach Worm) kills ghosts, evils, and ill matters. [Peach] grows in mountains and valleys.

---

[378] The current name of this medicinal is *Tao Ren*. It relaxes the liver, generates new blood, and drains stagnant blood. Hence it is able to treat blood accumulation due to falls and knocks, blood dysentery, blood block, heat penetrating the blood chamber, and cough with counterflow qi ascent. The following formulas containing Peach Seeds as a main ingredient were all designed by the medical sage, Zhang Zhong-jing (150-219 CE) and are still in wide use: *Tao Ren Cheng Qi Tang* (Peach Seed Order the Qi Decoction) treats blood amassment in the bladder giving rise to maniac illnesses. To treat blood accumulation, one may prescribe *Di Dang Tang* (Flushing Decoction). *Bie Jia Jian Wan* (Boiled Turtle Shell Pills) are a formula for hepatomegaly and splenomegaly. *Da Huang Mu Dan Pi Tang* (Rhubarb & Moutan Decoction) is effective for appendicitis.

In this passage, a number of things other than the seed are discussed, for instance, Peach Flower. However, in modern prescriptions, only Peach Seeds are often met and all the others are no longer used.

[379] This is peach fruit that has survived until winter on the tree.

Ku Piao (**Fructus Lagenariae Vulgaris**)[380] is bitter and cold. It mainly treats great water [giving rise to] puffy swelling of the face, eyes, and limbs. It precipitates water and makes one vomit. It grows in rivers and swamps.

Shui Jin (**Herba Oenanthis Javanicae**)[381] is sweet and balanced. It mainly treats red ooze in females, stops bleeding, nourishes the essence, protects the blood vessels, boosts the qi, and makes one fat, strong, and desirous of food. Its other name is *Shui Ying* (Water Flower). It grows in pools and swamps.

---

[380] Besides the indications listed in the text, Calabash or Bottle Gourd is said to be good for blood ejection, hemafecia, wasting thirst, stone strangury, roundworms, and malign sores. Nowadays, however, it is seldom used except for ascites.

[381] The current name is *Shui Qin*. Chen Cang-qi said, "The juice extracted from its leaves and stalk after they have been smashed is able to relieve sudden fever in children and hangover of heat toxins, nasal congestion, and generalized fever after having drunk as well as to disinhibit the large and small intestines."

Cereals: Superior Class

Hu Ma (**Semen Sesami Indicae**)[382] is sweet and balanced. It is nontoxic, mainly treating damaged center with vacuity and languor. It supplements the five internals, boosts the qi and [physical] force, promotes the growth of the muscles and flesh, and replenishes the brain marrow. Protracted taking may make the body light and prolong life. The leaf [Folium Sesami Indicae] is called *Qing Xiang*. [Sesame] is also called *Ju Sheng* (Major Triumph). It grows in rivers and valleys.

---

[382] Sesame supplements the lung qi, moistens the five viscera, replenishes the marrow, blackens the hair, expels wind dampness, and heals incised wounds and sores. In his annotation on this passage, Ye Gui said:

Yin is the guardian of the center. Damaged center is damaged yin blood. The lungs are the source of transformation of fluids, the spleen controls the blood, and the heart governs the blood. Sesame enters the spleen, lungs, and heart. It is sweet [in flavor] and balanced [of qi] and, therefore, boosts the blood. For that reason, it rules damaged center. The spleen governs the muscles and flesh. The sweet flavor moistens the spleen. Therefore, [Sesame] rules vacuity and emaciation. The five internals are inside the five viscera where yin is stored. Sesame is enriching and moistening. Therefore, it supplements the five viscera.

Because Sesame is able to supplement the lung qi, replenish the five viscera, and moisten the five viscera, it blackens the hair, dispels wind dampness, and heals incised wounds and sores. Sesame Oil is also a medicinal that is able to cool the blood and resolve toxins, relieve pain and promote the growth of the muscles [*i.e.*, flesh].

Ma Fen (**Herba Cannabis Sativae**)[383] is acrid and balanced. It mainly treats the seven damages, disinhibits the five viscera, and precipitates the blood and cold qi. Taking much of it may make one behold ghosts and frenetically run about. Protracted taking may enable one to communicate with the spirit light and make the body light. The seed [Semen Cannabis Sativae] is sweet and balanced. It mainly supplements the center and boosts the qi. Protracted taking may make one fat, strong, and never senile. [Herba Cannabis Sativae] is also called *Ma Bo* (Hemp Erection). It grows in rivers and valleys.

---

[383] The current name of this medicinal is *Da Ma*. Its seed is currently called *Ma Ren* or *Da Ma Ren*. In modern clinical practice, Hemp Seeds are still in wide use. They are able to dredge wind qi, relax the spleen, moisten dryness, promote lactation, hasten delivery, and disinhibit urination and defecation.

Cereals: Middle Class

Da Dou Huang Juan (Semen Germinatus Glycinis Hispidae)[384] is sweet and balanced. It is nontoxic, mainly treating damp impediment, sinew hypertonicity, and pain in the knee. *Sheng Da Dou* (uncooked Semen Glycinis Hispidae)[385] can be applied to abscesses and swellings. Its juice can be boiled. Drinking it may kill ghost toxins and relieve pain. *Chi Xiao*

---

[384] According to Tao Hong-jing, Soybean Sprouts are able to boost the qi, break binding in the five viscera and stomach, and resolve toxins. In addition, they are able to flush malign blood. In his annotation on this part, Zou Shu said that although there are many medicinals that are able to treat sinew cramps and hypertonicity, for example, *Mu Gua* (Fructus Chaenomelis Lagenariae), Coix, and Achyranthes, none of them are better than Soybean Sprouts.

[385] In olden times, Soybean Seeds seemed to be in wide use as medicinals. Tao Hong-jing said:

> They dispel water distention, eliminate heat impediment in the stomach, damaged center, and *lin lu* [exposure to dew], precipitate blood stasis, dissipate internal cold accumulation and binding in the five viscera, and resolve Aconite toxins... [In addition,] they eliminate swelling, remove impediment, disperse grain, and relieve abdominal distention.

However, they are seldom used in modern prescriptions.

Soybean juice or milk is prepared in the following way. First soak the beans overnight and then grind with water. After filtering, there is white juice or "milk" left. In North China, people drink this for breakfast.

Dou (Semen Phaseoli Calcarati)[386] mainly precipitates water and expels pus and blood from abscesses and swellings. They grow in plains and swamps.

Su Mi (**Semen Setariae**) is bitter. It is nontoxic, mainly nourishing the kidney qi, removing heat from the spleen and stomach, and boosting the qi. Stale [Setaria] is bitter. It mainly treats stomach heat and wasting thirst and disinhibits urination.

Shu Mi (**Semen Panici Miliacei**) is sweet. It is nontoxic, mainly boosting the qi, supplementing the center, and [relieving] abundant heat giving rise to vexation.

---

[386] Aduki Beans are sweet and sour in flavor and balanced of qi. Nowadays, they are mainly used to move water to disinhibit urination, dissipate the blood to disperse swelling, and clear heat to resolve toxins. They are, therefore, a good medicinal for hemafecia, water swelling, foot qi, blood dysentery, difficult or scanty lactation, and all sorts of sores.

Cereals: Inferior Class

Fu Bi (**Flos Phaseoli Calcarati**)[387] is acrid and balanced. It mainly treats malaria with cold and heat, evil qi, diarrhea, dysentery, impotence, and headache [due to] hangover from wine.

---

[387] Athough this medicinal is a flower, because it is derived from a plant whose main product is a major cereal, Mung Beans, it is classified under cereals, not under herbs.

Book Four

Omission[388] from the *Ben Cao Jing*

Superior class medicinals keep one fit and increase one's life span, enabling one to ascend to heaven to become an immortal who is then able to travel freely up and down, bossing all the spirits about. [This person] will grow feathers over their body and be able to order meals any time while travelling. Middle class medicinals cultivate temperament, while inferior class medicinals eliminate disease. These are able to ward off toxic insects and worms, hold back wild beasts, prevent malign qi from spreading, and keep off ill and demonic matters. Tai Yi Zi[389] said, "Of the medicinals, the superior class nourishes life, the middle helps temperament, and the inferior helps disease." The Divine Farmer made a red whip as a tool for

---

[388] This whole part, *i.e.*, Book Four, is not found in the Chinese version we have taken as the basis of this translation but is attached at the end of some other versions as a supplement. This is included even though the editors all knew that this part overlaps the text in some way. It should also be noted that most passages in this part were undoubtedly inserted by some later editors. In some versions, there are some passages headed by the words *Xu Li Bai Zi* (Preface Written in White) preceding this part. However, these passages are different from version to version.

[389] The words *tai yi* mean primal, archetypal, or supreme and are often used to refer to the supreme god or the beginning of the cosmos. The character *zi* is the title of a Daoist. Tai Yi Zi is the name of the assistant of the Divine Farmer. It seems that he acted in the same capacity as Qi Bo to the Yellow Emperor.

the investigation [of medicinals],[390] following the six yin and six yang.[391] He toured the five mountains and four rivers together with Tai Yi.[392] He made a study of each of the thousands of things the land produced—herbs, stones, bones, flesh, hearts, segments, skins, hairs, and feathers. [As a result,] he attained knowledge about what they could rule and their five flavors. Each day he was poisoned 70 times.[393] Bowing again, the Divine Farmer asked Tai Yi Zi, "(I) once heard that beyond a 100 years old, (people) become senile. What kind of qi is resposible for this?"

Tai Yi Zi answered, "There are nine entrances to the heaven. The middle one is the best." Then the Divine Farmer followed him [out through the middle entrance], going to taste medicinals to save the lives of the people.

Medicinals that have great toxins cannot be taken. Once a person takes them through the mouth, nose, ear, or eye, the person will be killed. The first [such medicinal] is *Gou Wen* (Gelsemium Elegans). The second is *Chi* (Circus Cyaneus). The third is *Yin Ming* (Yin Life).[394] The fourth is *Nei Tong*

---

[390] There is a legend that goes as follows. The Divine Farmer made a red whip and used it to whip the herbs he met. Thus he got to know their nature and flavors. Then he taught people how to grow plants and collect medicinals. This is how he acquired the title Divine Farmer.

[391] There are three yin and three yang channels in each of the arms and legs. Thus we have six yin channels and six yang channels.

[392] There are five holy mountains in China. They are Mount Tai in the east, Mount Hua in the west, Mount Song in the center, Mount Heng in the south, and Mount Heng in the north. The four rivers refer to the Yangtze, the Yellow, the Huai, and the Ji. The last one has long been a branch of the Yellow River.

[393] It was believed that the Divine Farmer tried to learn the uses of medicinals through tasting various herbs. Many times he was poisoned by some medicinals, but each time he saved himself by successfully discovering the other medicinals that might resolve the toxins.

[394] This is a lengendary animal. It is hard to tell its identity. There is a note under this passage saying that this is a red-colored animal which makes its nest in trees, hanging its baby on a tree and brooding it in the sea.

(Internal Child).[395] The fifth is *Zhen Yu* (Poisonous Feather).[396] The sixth is *Gao Xi* (Tall and Rare).[397]

There are five materials [that can resolve toxic] medicinals. First, *Lang Du* (Radix Galarhoei Eblactealati) can be resolved by *Zhan Si* (Cocoon of Monema Flavescens). Second, *Ba Tou* (Semen Crotonis Tiglii) can be resolved by *Huo Zhi* (Succus Agastachis Seu Pogostemi).[398] Third, *Li Lu* (Radix Et Rhizoma Veratri) can be resolved by soup.[399] Fourth, *Tian Xiong* (Radix Lateralis Aconiti Carmichaeli) and *Wu Tou* (Radix Aconiti) can be resolved by *Da Dou* (Semen Glycinis Hispidae). Fifth, *Ban Mao* (Mylabris) can be resolved by *Rong Yan* (Alkali). If poisonous vegetables have done harm to small children, one may resolve this by breast milk. First administer two *sheng*.

The five *Zhi* (Ganoderma), *Er Dan Sha* (Cinnabar), *Yu Zha* (Nephritum), *Ceng Qing* (Azuritum), *Xiong Huang* (Realgar), *Ci Huang* (Auripigmentum), *Yun Mu* (Muscovitum), and *Tai Yi Yu Yu Liang* (Limonitum) can each be administered singly. They may enable the taker to fly and enjoy longevity.

Spring and summer are yang, while autumn and winter are yin. Spring is yang, and yang warms and generates the tens of thousands of things.

---

[395] This is another legendary animal. There is a note under this passage saying that this looks like a goose and also broods its baby in the sea.

[396] This is yet another legendary animal. There is a note under this passage saying that this looks like a sparrow with a black head and red beak.

[397] This is again a lengendary animal. There is a note under this passage saying that it is born in the sea and that the male is called *xi*, while the female is called *gao*.

[398] Croton Seed can be poisonous. Its toxins can be resolved, however, by thin Mung Bean gruel or Soybean Juice.

[399] The toxins of Veratrum Root can be resolved by atropine or ephedrine. As a folk remedy, thick Chinese Scallion soup or a cold mixture of onion, Realgar, pig fat, and tea can also be used to resolve the toxins. However, the translator suspects that the word soup (*tang*) here simply means boiled water.

If one takes *Huang Jing* (Rhizoma Polygonati) and *Zhu* (Rhizoma Atractylodis), one may be able to fast on grain or can survive years of famine without grain. They are called grain substitutes.

The five flavors [*i.e.*, grains] nourish the essence spirit and fortify the ethereal and corporeal souls, while the five stones nourish the marrow and fatten and render luster to the muscles and flesh. Of the various medicinals, the sour flavored ones supplement the liver, nourish the heart, and eliminate kidney disease. The bitter flavored ones supplement the heart, nourish the spleen, and eliminate liver disease. The sweet flavored ones supplement the lungs, nourish the spleen, and eliminate heart disease. The acrid flavored ones supplement the lungs, nourish the kidneys, and eliminate spleen disease. The salty flavored ones supplement the lungs and eliminate liver disease. The five flavors correspond to the five phases, while the four limbs correspond to the four seasons. Personalities [are decided by] the four seasons in which people are born, and they accordingly correspond to the five phases. Supplementing the body with the primary[400] may make one immortal and ordain one a deity. Supplementing the child with the mother[400] may render longevity. The child protecting the mother[400] may eliminate disease and lengthen the life span.

---

[400] According to one's season of birth, one corresponds to one of the five phases. For example, one corresponds to fire if one is born in summer. In this case, medicinals corresponding to fire are referred to as primary and their flavor should be bitter. Taking bitter medicinals, the heart will be supplemented. Wood is the mother of fire. If the person takes sour flavored medicinals, this is the mother nourishing the child. If, on the contrary, the person takes sweet flavored medicinals corresponding to earth, this is the child protecting the mother. This is because the sweet flavor (earth) is the child of the bitter flavor (fire).

A Supplement of 12 Passages from Wu's *Ben Cao* (Wu's Materia Medica)[401]

Long Yan (Arillus Euphoriae Longanae) is also called *Yi Zhi* (Wits Sharpener). Yet another name is *Bi Mu* (Parallel Eyes).

Shu Wei (Fructus Piperis Longi) is also called *Jin* (Strength). Yet another name is *Shan Ling Qiao* (Hill's Prominence). It treats dysentery.

Pu Yin Shi (Fructus Elaeagni Pungentis) grows in plains and valleys or in gardens. [The tree] branches with leaves like the melon's and its fruit is like the peach. [The fruit] is collected in the seventh month. It quenches thirst and prolongs life.

Qian Sui Yuan (Old Wall Clay)[402] is good for the skin. It treats [the skin] together with *Jiang* (Rhizome Zingiberis) and *Chi Shi Zhi* (Hallyositum Rubrum).

Xiao Hua (Polygala Tenuifolia) is also called *Jie Cao* (Bind Weed).

Mu Gua (Fructus Chaenomelis Lagenariae) grows in Yi Ling.[403]

---

[401] Wu was the surname of Wu Pu who was a pupil of the most distinguished physician, Hua Tuo. His materia medica, which has long been lost, was supposed to be based on the *Sheng Nong Ben Cao Jing*.

[402] This identification is questionable.

[403] This is a place in the present-day Hubei Province.

Gu Shu Pi (Cortex Ailanthi Altissimi) treats throat block. Its other name is *Chu*.

Ying Tao (Fructus Pruni Pseudocerasi) is sweet. It mainly regulates the center and boosts the qi, renders the facial complexion attractive, and glorifies the will qi.[404] Its other name is *Zhu Tao* (Vermilion Peach). Yet another name is *Mai Ying* (Wheat Flower).

Li He (Semen Pruni) treats collapse. The flower [Flos Pruni] may render the facial complexion attractive.

Da Mai (Semen Hordei Vulgaris) is also called *Kuang Mai* (Broad Wheat). It is the most exuberant [*i.e.*, richest] of all the five grains. It is nontoxic, treating wasting thirst, eliminating heat, and boosting the qi. *Shi Mi* (Honey) is its envoy. *Mai Zhong* (Semen Tritici) is also called *Xiao Mai* (Small Wheat). It is nontoxic, treating dysentery but is not good for [blank].[405]

Chi (Semen Praeparatus Sojae) boosts people's qi.

Hui Ri (Bright Sun)[406] is also called *Zhen Yu* (Poisonous Bird Feather).

---

[404] In ancient times, medicinals were believed not only to remedy disease but also to improve the personality and temperament. The word *zhi qi* (will qi), if translated freely, means ambition or aspiration. See Note 1, Fruits & Vegetables: Middle Class, Book III.

[405] There is a word missing here.

[406] This is a mythical bird whose feathers are said to be fatally poisonous.

A Supplement: Restrainers and Envoys of Various Medicinals

Jades and Stones: Superior Class

Yu Quan (Nephritum) fears *Kuan Dong Hua* (Flos Tussilaginis Farfarae).

Yu Xie (Nephritum Powder) is averse to *Lu Jiao* (Cornu Cervi).

Dan Sha (Cinnabar) is averse to *Ci Shi* (Magnetitum) and fears *Jian Shui* (Alkali).

Ceng Qing (Azuritum) fears *Tu Si Zi* (Semen Cuscutae Chinensis).

The envoy of *Shi Dan* (Chalcabthitum) is *Shui Ying* (Herba Oenanthis Javanicae). It fears *Mu Gui* (Cortex Cinnamomi Cassiae), *Jun Gui* (tubiform Cortex Cinnamomi Cassiae), *Yuan Hua* (Flos Daphnis Genkwae), and *Xin Yi Bai* (Flos Albi Magnoliae Liliflorae).

The envoy of *Zhong Ru* (Stalactitum) is *She Chuang Zi* (Fructus Cnidii Monnieri). It is averse to *Mu Dan* (Cortex Radicis Moutan), *Mu Meng* (Radix Et Rhizoma Paridis Tetraphyllae), *Yuan Shi* (Magnititum), and *Mu Meng* (Radix Et Ehizoma Paridis Tetraphyllae)[sic], and fears *Zi Shi Ying* (Flouritum) and *Rang Cao* (Folium Zingiberis Miogae).

The envoy of *Yun Mu* (Muscovitum) is *Ze Xie* (Rhizoma Alismatis). It fears *Tuo Jia* (Squama Alligatoris Sinensis) and running water.

159

The envoy of *Xiao Shi* (Niter) is [blank].[407] It is averse to *Ku Shen* (Radix Sophorae Flavescentis) and *Ku Cai* (Herba Sonchi Olercei) and fears *Nu Wan* (Herba Asteris Fastigiati).

Po Xiao (Slaked Lime) fears *Mai Ju Jiang* (Herba Carpensii Abrotanoidis).

The envoy of *Mang Xiao* (Mirabilitum) is *Shi Wei* (Folium Pyrrosiae Linguae). It is averse to *Mai Ju Jiang* (Herba Carpensii Abrotanoidis).

The envoy of *Fan Shi* (Alumen) is *Gan Cao* (Radix Glycyrrhizae). It fears *Mu Li* (Concha Ostreae).

The envoy of *Hua Shi* (Talcum) is *Shi Wei* (Folium Pyrrosiae Linguae). It is averse to *Ceng Qing* (Azuritum).

The envoy of *Zi Shi Ying* (Flouritum) is *Chang Shi* (Anhydritum). It fears *Bian Qing* (Azuritum) and *Fu Zi* (Radix Lateralis Aconiti Carmichaeli) and is not partial to *Tuo Jia* (Squama Alligatoris Sinensis), *Huang Lian* (Rhizoma Coptidis Chinensis), and *Mai Ju Jiang* (Herba Carpensii Abrotanoidis).

Bai Shi Ying (Quartz Crystal) is averse to *Ma Mu* (Oculus Equus) and *Du Gong* (Radix Aconiti).

Chi Shi Zhi (Hallyositum Rubrum) is averse to *Da Huang* (Radix Et Rhizoma Rhei) and fears *Yuan Hua* (Flos Daphnis Genkwae).

The envoy of *Huang Shi Zhi* (Hallyositum Aureum) is *Ceng Qing* (Azuritum). It is averse to *Xi Xin* (Herba Asari Cum Radice) and fears *Fei Lian* (Stylopyga Conucina).

The envoy of *Tai Yi Yu Yu Liang* (Limonitum) is *Du Zhong* (Cortex Eucommiae Ulmoidis). It fears *Tie Luo* (Frusta Ferri), *Chang Pu* (Rhizoma Acori Graminei), and *Bei Mu* (Bulbus Fritillariae).

---

[407] The word missing here may be fire.

Jades and Stones: Middle Class

Shui Yin (Mercurius) fears *Ci Shi* (Magnetitum).

Yin Nie (Stalactitum) is averse to *Fang Ji* (Radix Stephaniae Tetrandrae) and fears *Mu* (Wood).

The envoy of *Kong Gong Nie* (Stalactitum) is *Mu Lan* (Cortex Magnoliae Liliflorae). It is averse to *Xi Xin* (Herba Asari Cum Radice).

The envoy of *Yang Qi Shi* (Actinolitum) is *Sang Piao Xiao* (Ootheca Mantidis). It is averse to *Ze Xie* (Rhizoma Alismatis), *Jun Gui* (tubiform Cortex Cinnamomi Cassiae), *Lei Wan* (Fructificatio Polypori Mylittae), and *She Tui Pi* (Exuviae Serpentis), and it fears *Tu Si Zi* (Semen Cuscutae Chinensis).

The envoy of *Shi Gao* (Gypsum) is *Ji Zi* (Chicken Egg). It is averse to *Mang Cao* (Folium Illicii Lanceolati) and *Du Gong* (Radix Aconiti).

Ning Shui Shi (Polyhalitum) fears *Di Yu* (Radix Sanguisorbae Officinalis). It resolves the toxins of *Ba Dou* (Semen Crotonis Tiglii).

The envoy of *Ci Shi* (Magnetitum) is *Chai Hu* (Radix Bupleuri). It fears *Huang Shi Zhi* (Hallyositum Aureum) and is averse to *Mu Dan* (Cortex Radicis Moutan) and *Mang Cao* (Folium Illicii Lanceolati).

Yuan Shi (Magnetitum Atrum) is averse to *Song Zhi* (Resina Pini), *Bai Zi Ren* (Semen Biotae Orientalis), and *Jun Gui* (tubiform Cortex Cinnamomi Cassiae).

The envoy of *Li Shi* (Gypsum Fibrosum) is *Hua Shi* (Talcum). It is averse to *Ma Huang* (Herba Ephedrae).

161

Jades and Stones: Inferior Class

Fan Shi (Alumen) will become better if it acquires fire. Its envoy is *Ji Zhen* (Spina Zizyphi Jujubae). It is averse to *Hu Zhang* (Rhizoma Polygoni Cuspidati), *Du Gong* (Radix Aconiti), *Wu Shi* (Feces Anatis Domesticae), *Xi Xin* (Herba Asari Cum Radice), and water.

Qing Lang Gan (Malachitum) will become better if it acquires *Shui Yin* (Mercurius). It fears *Ji Gu* (Os Galli Galli) and kills the toxins of *Xi* (Tin).

Te Sheng Fan Shi (Alum) will become better if it acquires fire. It fears water.

Dai Zhe (Haemititum) fears *Tian Xiong* (Radix Lateralis Aconiti Carmichaeli).

Fang Jie Shi (Calcitum) is averse to *Ba Dou* (Semen Crotonis Tiglii).

The envoy of *Da Yan* (Sal) is *Lou Lu* (Radix Echinponsis Seu Rhapontici).

Herbs: Superior Class

The envoy of *Liu Zhi* (The Six Species of Ganoderma) is *Shu Yu* (Rhizoma Dioscoreae Oppositae). They will become better if they acquire *Fa* (Crinis Humanis). They are averse to *Chang Shan* (Radix Dichroae Febrifugae) and fear *Bian Qing* (Azuritum) and *Yin Chen* (Herba Artemisiae Capillaris).

The envoys of *Zhu* (Rhizoma Atractylodis) are *Fang Feng* (Radix Ledebouriellae Divaricatae) and *Di Yu* (Radix Sanguisorbae Officinalis).

The envoys of *Tian Men Dong* (Tuber Asparagi Cochinensis) are *Yuan Yi* (Herba Bryi Argenti) and *Di Huang* (Radix Rehmanniae). It fears *Ceng Qing* (Azuritum).

The envoys of *Mai Men Dong* (Tuber Ophiopogonis Japonici) are *Di Huang* (Radix Rehmanniae) and *Che Qian* (Semen Plantaginis). It is averse to *Kuan*

Dong (Flos Tussilaginis Farfarae) and *Ku Piao* (Fructus Lagenariae Sicerariae), and it fears *Ku Shen* (Radix Sophorae Flavescentis) and *Qing Xiang* (Semen Celosiae Argenteae).

Nu Wei Rui (Rhizoma Polygonati Odorati) mainly fears *Lu Shi Yan* (Alkali).

Gan Di Huang (dry Radix Rehmanniae) will become better if it acquires *Mai Men Dong* (Tuber Ophiopogonis Japonici) and clear wine [*i.e.*, alcohol]. It is averse to *Bei Mu* (Bulbus Fritillariae) and fears *Wu Yi* (Semen Praeparatus Ulmi Macrocarpae).

The envoys of *Chang Pu* (Rhizoma Acori Graminei) are *Qin Hua* (Flos Fraxini) and *Qin Pi* (Cortex Fraxini). It is averse to *Di Dan* (Meloe Coartatus) and *Ma Huang* (Herba Ephedrae).

Ze Xie (Rhizoma Alismatis) fears *Hai Ge* (Concha Cyclinae Sinensis) and *Wen Ge* (Concha Cythirae Meretricis).

Yuan Zhi (Radix Polygalae Tenuifoliae) will become better if it acquires *Fu Ling* (Sclerotium Poriae Cocos), *Dong Kui Zi* (Semen Abutili Seu Malvae), and *Long Gu* (Os Draconis). It kills the toxins of *Tian Xiong* (Radix Lateralis Aconiti Carmichaeli) and *Fu Zi* (Radix Lateralis Aconiti Carmichaeli). It fears *Zhen Zhu* (Margarita), *Fei Lian* (Stylopyga Conucina), and *Li Lu* (Radix Et Rhizoma Veratri).

The envoys of *Qi Ge* (Mactra Quandrangularis) are *Shu Yu* (Radix Dioscoreae Oppositae) and *Zi Zhi* (Ganoderma Purpurea). It is averse to *Gan Sui* (Radix Euphobiae Kansui).

The envoy of *Shi Jie* (Radix Stephaniae Tetrandae) is *Lu Ying* (Flos Sambuci Javanicae). It is averse to *Ning Shui Shi* (Polyhalitum) and *Ba Dou* (Semen Crotonis Tiglii), and it fears *Bai Jiang Can* (Bombyx Batryticatus) and *Lei Wan* (Fructificatio Polypori Mylittae).

The envoys of *Ju Hua* (Flos Chrysanthemi Morifolii) are *Zhu* (Rhizoma Atractylodis), *Gou Qi Gen* (Radix Lycii Chinensis), and *Sang Gen Bai Pi* (Cortex Radicis Mori Albi).

163

The envoys of *Gan Cao* (Radix Glycyrrhizae) are *Zhu* (Rhizoma Atractylodis), *Gan Qi* (Lacca Sinica Exsiccata), and *Ku Shen* (Radix Sophorae Flavescentis). It is averse to *Yuan Zhi* (Radix Polygalae Tenuifoliae) and clashes with *Gan Sui* (Radix Euphorbiae Kansui), *Da Ji* (Herba Seu Radix Cirsii Japonici), *Yuan Hua* (Flos Daphnis Genkwae), and *Hai Zao* (Herba Sargassii).

The envoy of *Ren Shen* (Radix Panacis Ginseng) is *Fu Ling* (Sclerotium Poriae Cocos). It is averse to *Sou Shu* (Semen Deutziae Scabrae) and clashes with *Li Lu* (Radix Et Rhizoma Veratri).

Niu Xi (Radix Achyranthis Bidentatae) is averse to *Ying Huo Chong* (Luciola Vitticollis) and *Lu Ying* (Flos Sambuci Javanicae) and it fears the white.

The envoys of *Xi Xin* (Herba Asari Cum Radice) are *Ceng Qing* (Azuritum) and *Dong Gen* (Rhizoma Anemarrhenae Asphodeloidis). It is averse to *Lang Du* (Radix Stellerae Chamaejasmis), *Shan Zhu Yu* (Fructus Corni Officinalis), and *Huang Qi* (Radix Astragali Membranacei). It fears *Hua Shi* (Talcum) and *Xiao Shi* (Niter), and it clashes with *Li Lu* (Radix Et Rhizoma Veratri).

The envoy of *Du Huo* (Radix Angelicae Pubescentis) is *Li Shi* (Gypsum Fibrosum).

The envoy of *Chai Hu* (Radix Bupleuri) is *Ban Xia* (Rhizoma Pinelliae Ternatae). It is averse to *Zao Jia* (Fructus Gleditschiae Chinensis) and fears *Nu Wan* (Radix Asteris Fastigiati) and *Li Lu* (Radix Et Rhizoma Veratri).

The envoys of *An Lu Zi* (Fructus Artemisiae Keiskeanae) are *Jing Zi* (Fructus Viticis) and *Yi Yi Ren* (Semen Coicis Lachryma-jobi).

Xi Ming Zi (Semen Thlaspi Arvensis) will become better if it acquires *Jing Zi* (Fructus Viticis) and *Xi Xin* (Herba Asari Cum Radice). It is averse to *Gan Jiang* (dry Rhizoma Zingiberis) and *Ku Shen* (Radix Sophorae Flavescentis).

The envoy of *Long Dan* (Radix Gentianae Scabrae) is *Guan Zhong* (Rhizoma Dryopteridis). It is averse to *Fang Kui* (Radix Peucedani Japonici) and *Di Huang* (Radix Rehmanniae).

Tu Si Zi (Semen Cuscutae Chinensis) will become better if it acquires wine. Its envoys are *Shu Yu* (Radix Dioscoreae Oppositae) and *Song Zhi* (Resina Pini). It is averse to *Huan Jun* (Herba Phragmitis Communis).

The envoy of *Ba Ji Tian* (Radix Morindae Officinalis) is *Fu Pen Zi* (Fructus Rubi Chingii). It is averse to *Zhao Sheng* (Coprinus Atramentarius), *Lei Wan* (Fructificatio Polypori Mylittae), and *Dan Shen* (Radix Salviae Miltiorrhizae).

The envoy of *Ji Li Zi* (Semen Astragali Complanati) is *Wu Tou* (Radix Aconiti).

Sha Shen (Radix Glehniae Littoralis) is averse to *Fang Ji* (Radix Stephaniae Tetrandrae) and clashes with *Li Lu* (Radix Et Rhizoma Veratri).

Fang Feng (Radix Ledebouriellae Divaricatae) is averse to *Gan Jiang* (dry Rhizoma Zingiberis), *Li Lu* (Radix Et Rhizoma Veratri), *Bai Lian* (Radix Ampelopsis Japonicae), and *Yuan Hua* (Flos Daphnis Genkwae). It kills the toxins of *Fu Zi* (Radix Lateralis Aconiti Carmichaeli).

The envoys of *Luo Shi* (Folium Trachelospermi Jasminoidis) are *Du Zhong* (Cortex Eucommiae Ulmoidis) and *Mu Dan* (Cortex Radicis Moutan). It is averse to *Tie Luo* (Frusta Ferri) and fears *Chang Pu* (Rhizoma Acori Graminei) and *Bei Mu* (Bulbus Fritillariae).

The envoys of *Huang Lian* (Rhizoma Coptidis Chinensis) are *Huang Qin* (Radix Scutellariae Baicalensis), *Long Gu* (Os Drconis), and *Li Shi* (Gypsum Fibrosum). It is averse to *Ju Hua* (Flos Chrysanthemi Morifolii), *Yuan Hua* (Flos Daphnis Genkwae), *Yuan Shen* (Radix Scrophulariae Ningpoensis), and *Bai Xian Pi* (Cortex Radicis Dictamni Dasycarpi). It fears *Kuan Dong* (Flos Tussilaginis Farfarae), restrains *Wu Tou* (Radix Aconiti), and resolves the toxins of *Ba Dou* (Semen Crotonis Tiglii).

Dan Shen (Radix Salviae Miltiorrhizae) fears *Yan Shui* (Alkali) and clashes with *Li Lu* (Radix Et Rhizoma Veratri).

The envoy of *Tian Ming Jing* (Herba Carpensii Abrotanoides) is *Yuan Yi* (Herba Bryi Argenti).

The envoy of *Jue Ming Zi* (Semen Cassiae Torae) is *Chu Shi* (Fructus Achilleae Alpinae). It is averse to *Da Ma Zi* (Semen Cannabis Sativae).

The envoy of *Xu Duan* (Radix Dipsaci) is *Di Huang* (Radix Rehmanniae). It is averse to *Lei Wan* (Fructificatio Polypori Mylittae).

The envoy of *Xiong Qiong* (Radix Ligustici Wallichii) is *Bai Zhi* (Radix Angelicae Dahuricae).

Huang Qi (Radix Astragali Membranacei) is averse to *Gui Jia* (Plastrum Testudinis).

Du Ruo (Herba Polliae Japonicae) will become better if it acquires *Xin Yi* (Flos Magnoliae Liliflorae) and *Xi Xin* (Herba Asari Cum Radice). It is averse to *Chai Hu* (Radix Bupleuri) and *Qian Hu* (Radix Peucedani).

She Chuang Zi (Fructus Cnidii Monnieri) is averse to *Mu Dan* (Cortex Radicis Moutan), *Ba Dou* (Semen Crotonis Tiglii), and *Bei Mu* (Bulbus Fritillariae).

Qian Gen (Radix Rubiae Cordifoliae) fears *Shu Gu* (Cortex Radicis Moutan).

Fei Lian (Herba Carduus Crispi) will become better if it acquires *Wu Tou* (Radix Aconiti). It is averse to *Ma Huang* (Herba Ephedrae).

Wei Xin (Herba Gnaphalii Affineae) will become better if it acquires *Qin Pi* (Cortex Fraxini).

The envoy of *Wu Wei Zi* (Fructus Schisandrae Chinensis) is *Cong Rong* (Herba Cistanchis Deserticolae). It is averse to *Wei Rui* (Rhizoma Polygonati Odorati) and restrains *Wu Tou* (Radix Aconiti).

Herbs: Middle Class

Dang Gui (Radix Angelicae Sinensis) is averse to *Lu Ru* (Radix Euphorbiae Adenochlorae) and fears *Chang Pu* (Rhizoma Acori Graminei), *Hai Zao* (Herba Sargassii), and *Mu Meng* (Radix Et Ehizoma Paridis Tetraphyllae).

The envoy of *Qin Jiao* (Radix Gentianae Macrophyllae) is *Chang Pu* (Rhizoma Acori Graminei).

The envoys of *Huang Qin* (Radix Scutellariae Baicalensis) are *Shan Zhu Yu* (Fructus Corni Officinalis) and *Long Gu* (Os Draconis). It is averse to *Cong Shi* (Semen Allii Fistulosi) and fears *Dan Sha* (Cinnabar), *Mu Dan* (Cortex Radicis Moutan), and *Li Lu* (Radix Et Rhizoma Veratri).

The envoy of *Shao Yao* (Radix Paeoniae Lactiflorae) is *Xu Wan* (Hematitum). It is averse to *Shi Hu* (Herba Dendrobii) and *Mang Xiao* (Mirabilitum), fears *Shi Bie Jia* (fossilized Plastrum Chitonis) and *Xiao Ji* (Herba Cephalanoplos Segeti), and clashes with *Li Lu* (Radix Et Rhizoma Veratri).

The envoy of *Gan Jiang* (dry Rhizoma Zingiberis) is *Qin Jiao* (Pericarpium Zanthoxyli Bungeani). It is averse to *Huang Lian* (Rhizoma Coptidis Chinensis), *Huang Qin* (Radix Scutellariae Baicalensis), and *Tian Shu Shi* (Excrementum Verpertilionis Murini), and kills the toxins of *Ban Xia* (Rhizoma Pinelliae Ternatae) and *Lang Dang* (Semen Scopoliae Japonicae).

Gao Ben (Radix Et Rhizoma Ligustici Chinensis) fears *Lu Ru* (Radix Euphorbiae Adenochlorae).

Th envoy of *Ma Huang* (Herba Ephedrae) is *Hou Po* (Cortex Magnoliae Officinalis). It is averse to *Xin Yi* (Flos Magnoliae Liliflorae) and *Shi Wei* (Folium Pyrrosiae Linguae).

167

Ge Gen (Radix Puerariae) kills the toxins of *Ye Ge* (Herba Gelsemii Elegantis), *Ba Dou* (Semen Crotonis Tiglii), and hundreds of [other] medicinals.

The envoy of *Qian Hu* (Radix Peucedani) is *Ban Xia* (Rhizoma Pinelliae Ternatae). It is averse to *Zao Jia* (Fructus Gleditschiae Chinensis) and fears *Li Lu* (Radix Et Rhizoma Veratri).

The envoys of *Bei Mu* (Bulbus Fritillariae) are *Hou Po* (Cortex Magnoliae Officinalis) and *Bai Wei* (Radix Cynanchi Baiwei). It is averse to *Tao Hua* (Flos Pruni Persicae), fears *Qin Jiao* (Radix Gentianae Macrophyllae), *Fan Shi* (Alumen), and *Mang Cao* (Folium Illicii Lanceolati), and clashes with *Wu Tou* (Radix Aconiti).

The envoy of *Gua Lou* (Fructus Trichosanthis Kirlowii) is *Gou Qi* (Fructus Lycii Chinensis). It is averse to *Gan Jiang* (dry Rhizoma Zingiberis), fears *Niu Xi* (Radix Achyranthis Bidentatae) and *Gan Qi* (Lacca Sinica Exsiccata), and clashes with *Wu Tou* (Radix Aconiti).

Yuan Shen (Radix Scrophulariae Ningpoensis) is averse to *Huang Qi* (Radix Astragali Membranacei), *Gan Jiang* (dry Rhizoma Zingiberis), *Da Zao* (Fructus Zizyphi Jujubae), and *Shan Zhu Yu* (Fructus Corni Officinalis), and it clashes with *Li Lu* (Radix Et Rhizoma Veratri).

The envoy of *Ku Shen* (Radix Sophorae Flavescentis) is *Yuan Shen* (Radix Scrophulariae Ningpoensis). It is averse to *Bei Mu* (Bulbus Fritillariae), *Lou Lu* (Radix Echinponsis Seu Rhapontici), and *Tu Si Zi* (Semen Cuscutae Chinensis), and it clashes with *Li Lu* (Radix Et Rhizoma Veratri).

The envoy of *Shi Long Rui* (Herba Ranuculi Sclerati) is *Da Ji* (Herba Seu Radix Cirsii Japonici). It fears *She Tui* (Exuviae Serpentis) and *Wu Zhu Yu* (Fructus Evodiae Rutecarpae).

The envoy of *Bei Xie* (Rhizoma Dioscoreae Hypoglaucae) is *Yi Yi Ren* (Semen Coicis Lachryma-jobi). It fears *Kui Gen* (Radix Abutilonis Seu Malvae), *Da Huang* (Radix Et Rhizoma Rhei), *Chai Hu* (Radix Bupleuri), *Mu Li* (Concha Ostreae), and *Qian Hu* (Radix Peucedani).

The envoys of *Shi Wei* (Folium Pyrrosiae Linguae) are *Hua Shi* (Talcum) and *Xing Ren* (Semen Pruni Armeniacae). It will become better if it acquires *Chang Pu* (Rhizoma Acori Graminei).

The envoy of *Gou Ji* (Rhizoma Cibotii Barometsis) is *Bei Xie* (Rhizoma Dioscoreae Hypoglaucae). It is averse to *Bai Jiang* (Herba Patriniae Heterophyllae Cum Radice).

The envoys of *Qu Mai* (Herba Dianthi) are *Rang Cao* (Folium Zingiberis Miogae) and *Mu Dan* (Cortex Radicis Moutan). It is averse to *Piao Xiao* (Os Sepiae Seu Sepiellae).

The envoy of *Bai Zhi* (Radix Angelicae Dahuricae) is *Dang Gui* (Radix Angelicae Sinensis). It is averse to *Xuan Fu Hua* (Flos Inulae).

The envoy of *Zi Wan* (Radix Asteris Tatarici) is *Kuan Dong* (Flos Tussilaginis Farfarae). It is averse to *Tian Xiong* (Radix Lateralis Aconiti Carmichaeli), *Qu Mai* (Herba Dianthi), *Lei Wan* (Fructificatio Polypori Mylittae), and *Yuan Zhi* (Radix Polygalae Tenuifoliae), and it fears *Yin Chen* (Herba Artemisiae Capillaris).

Bai Xian Pi (Cortex Radicis Dictamni Dasycarpi) is averse to *Piao Xiao* (Os Sepiae Seu Sepiellae), *Jie Geng* (Radix Platycodi Grandiflori), *Fu Ling* (Sclerotium Poriae Cocos), and *Bei Xie* (Rhizoma Dioscoreae Hypoglaucae).

Bai Wei (Radix Cynanchi Baiwei) is averse to *Huang Qi* (Radix Astragali Membranacei), *Da Huang* (Radix Et Rhizoma Rhei), *Da Ji* (Herba Seu Radix Cirsii Japonici), *Gan Jiang* (dry Rhizoma Zingiberis), *Gan Qi* (Lacca Sinica Exsiccata), *Da Zao* (Fructus Zizyphi Jujubae), and *Shan Zhu Yu* (Fructus Corni Officinalis).

Zi Shen (Herba Salviae Chinensis) fears *Xin Yi* (Flos Magnoliae Liliflorae).

The envoy of *Yin Yang Huo* (Herba Epimedii) is *Shu Yu* (Radix Dioscoreae Oppositae).

The envoy of *Kuan Dong Hua* (Flos Tussilaginis Farfarae) is *Xing Ren* (Semen Pruni Armeniacae). It will become better if it acquires *Zi Wan* (Radix Asteris Tatarici). It is averse to *Zao Jia* (Fructus Gleditschiae Chinensis), *Xiao Shi* (Niter), and *Yuan Shen* (Radix Scrophulariae Ningpoensis), and it fears *Bei Mu* (Bulbus Fritillariae), *Xin Yi* (Flos Magnoliae Liliflorae), *Ma Huang* (Herba Ephedrae), *Huang Qin* (Radix Scutellariae Baicalensis), *Huang Lian* (Rhizoma Coptidis Chinensis), *Huang Qi* (Radix Astragali Membranacei), and *Qing Xiang* (Semen Celosiae Argenteae).

Mu Dan (Cortex Radicis Moutan) fears *Tu Si Zi* (Semen Cuscutae Chinensis).

The envoy of *Fang Ji* (Radix Stephaniae Tetrandrae) is *Yin Nie* (Stalactitum). It is averse to *Xi Xin* (Herba Asari Cum Radice), fears *Bei Xie* (Rhizoma Dioscoreae Hypoglaucae), and kills the toxins of *Xiong Huang* (Realgar).

Nu Wan (Radix Asteris Fastigiati) fears *Lu Yan* (Alkali).

The envoy of *Ze Lan* (Herba Lycopi Lucidi) is *Fang Ji* (Radix Stephaniae Tetrandrae).

Di Yu (Radix Sanguisorbae Officinalis) will become better if it acquires *Fa* (Crinis Humanis). It is averse to *Mai Men Dong* (Tuber Ophiopogonis Japonici).

Hai Zao (Herba Sargassi) clashes with *Gan Cao* (Radix Glycyrrhizae).

Herbs: Inferior Class

The envoy of *Da Huang* (Radix Et Rhizoma Rhei) is *Huang Qin* (Radix Scutellariae Baicalensis).

The envoy of *Jie Geng* (Radix Platycodi Grandiflori) is *Jie Pi* (Cortex Chrysanthemi Morifolii). It fears *Bai Ji* (Rhizoma Bletillae Striatae) and clashes with *Long Dan* (Radix Gentianae Scabrae) and *Long Yan* (Arillus Euphoriae Longanae).

The envoy of *Gan Sui* (Radix Euphorbiae Kansui) is *Gua Di* (Pediculus Curcumeris). It is averse to *Yuan Zhi* (Radix Polygalae Tenuifoliae) and clashes with *Gan Cao* (Radix Glycyrrhizae).

The envoy of *Ting Li* (Semen Lepidii Seu Descurainiae) is *Yu Pi* (Cortex Ulmi Pumilae). It will become better if it acquires wine, but it is averse to *Jiang Can* (Bombyx Batryticatus) and *Shi Long Rui* (Herba Ranuculi Sclerati).

The envoy of *Yuan Hua* (Flos Daphnis Genkwae) is *Jue Ming* (Semen Cassiae Torae). It clashes with *Gan Cao* (Radix Glycyrrhizae).

The envoy of *Ze Qi* (Herba Euphorbiae Helioscopiae) is *Xiao Dou* (Semen Phaseoli Calcarati). It is averse to *Shu Yu* (Radix Dioscoreae Oppositae).

Da Ji (Herba Seu Radix Cirsii Japonici) clashes with *Gan Cao* (Radix Glycyrrhizae).

The envoy of *Gou Wen* (Herba Gelsemii Elegantis) is *Ban Xia* (Rhizoma Pinelliae Ternatae). It is averse to *Huang Qin* (Radix Scutellariae Baicalensis).

The envoy of *Li Lu* (Radix Et Rhizoma Veratri) is *Huang Lian* (Rhizoma Coptidis Chinensis). It clashes with *Xi Xin* (Herba Asari Cum Radice), *Shao Yao* (Radix Paeoniae Lactiflorae), and *Wu Shen* (the Five *Shen, i.e.,* Radix Panacis Ginseng, Radix Salviae Miltiorrhizae, Radix Glehniae Littoralis, Radix Scrophulariae Ningpoensis, and Radix Pseustellariae Heterophyllae). It is averse to *Da Huang* (Radix Et Rhizoma Rhei).

The envoy of *Wu Tou Wu Hui* (Radix Aconiti) is *Mang Cao* (Folium Illicii Lanceolati). It clashes with *Ban Xia* (Rhizoma Pinelliae Ternatae), *Gua Lou* (Fructus Trichosanthis Kirlowii), *Bei Mu* (Bulbus Fritillariae), *Bai Lian* (Radix Ampelopsis Japonicae), and *Bai Ji* (Rhizoma Bletillae Striatae). It is averse to *Li Lu* (Radix Et Rhizoma Veratri).

171

The envoy of *Tian Xiong* (Radix Lateralis Aconiti Carmichaeli) is *Yuan Zhi* (Radix Polygalae Tenuifoliae). It is averse to *Fu Bi* (Flos Phaseoli Calcarati).

The envoy of *Fu Zi* (Radix Lateralis Aconiti Carmichaeli) is *Di Dan* (Meloe Coartatus). It is averse to *Wu Gong* (Scolopendra Subspinipes) and it fears *Fang Feng* (Radix Ledebouriellae Divaricatae), *Gan Cao* (Radix Glycyrrhizae), *Huang Qi* (Radix Astragali Membranacei), *Ren Shen* (Radix Panacis Ginseng), *Wu Jiu* (Cortex Radicis Sapii Sebiferi), and *Da Dou* (Semen Sojae).

The envoy of *Guan Zhong* (Rhizoma Dryopteridis) is *Huan Jun* (Herba Phragmitis Communis).

The envoy of *Ban Xia* (Rhizoma Pinelliae Ternatae) is *She Gan* (Rhizoma Belamcandae Chinensis). It is averse to *Zao Jia* (Fructus Gleditschiae Chinensis), fears *Xiong Huang* (Realgar), *Sheng Jiang* (uncooked Rhizoma Zingiberis), *Gan Jiang* (dry Rhizoma Zingiberis), *Qin Pi* (Cortex Fraxini), and *Gui Jia* (Plastrum Testudinis), and clashes with *Wu Tou* (Radix Aconiti).

The envoy of *Shu Qi* (Folium Et Ramulus Dichroae Febrifugae) is *Gua Lou* (Fructus Trichosanthis Kirlowii). It is averse to *Guan Zhong* (Rhizoma Dryopteridis).

The envoy of *Hu Zhang* (Rhizoma Polygoni Cuspidati) is *Shu Qi* (Folium Et Ramulus Dichroae Febrifugae). It is averse to *Mang Cao* (Folium Illicii Lanceolati).

The envoy of *Lang Ya* (Herba Agrimoniae Pilosae) is *Wu Yi* (Semen Praeparatus Ulmi Macrocarpae). It is averse to *Zao Ji* (Fructus Cnidii Monnieri) and *Di Yu* (Radix Sanguisorbae Officinalis).

Chang Shan (Radix Dichroae Febrifugae) fears *Yu Zha* (Nephritum).

The envoy of *Bai Ji* (Rhizoma Bletillae Striatae) is *Zi Shi Ying* (Flouritum). It is averse to *Li Shi* (Gypsum Fibrosum), *Li He Ren* (Semen Pruni), and *Xing Ren* (Semen Pruni Armeniacae).

The envoy of *Bai Lian* (Radix Ampelopsis Japonicae) is *Dai Zhe* (Haemititum). It clashes with *Wu Tou* (Radix Aconiti).

Huan Jun (Herba Phragmitis Communis) will become better if it acquires wine. It fears *Ji Zi* (Chicken Egg).

The envoy of *Lu Ru* (Radix Euphorbiae Adenochlorae) is *Gan Cao* (Radix Glycyrrhizae). It is averse to *Mai Men Dong* (Tuber Ophiopogonis Japonici).

Jin Cao (Herba Arthrixi Hispidi) fears *Shu Fu* (Armadillidium Vulgare).

The envoy of *Xia Ku Cao* (Spica Prunellae Vulgaris) is *Tu Gua* (Fructus Trichosanthis Cucummeroidis).

The envoy of *Lang Du* (Radix Stellerae Chamaejasmes) is *Da Dou* (Semen Glycinis Hispidae). It is averse to *Mai Ju Jiang* (Herba Carpensii Abrotanoidis).

Gui Jiu (Rhizoma Dysosmae Versipellis) fears *Yi* (Herba Bryi Argenti).

Woods: Superior Class

The envoy of *Fu Ling* (Sclerotium Poriae Cocos) and *Fu Shen* (Sclerotium Pararadicis Poriae Cocos) is *Ma Xian* (Herba Pedicularis Resupinatae). They are averse to *Bai Lian* (Radix Ampelopsis Japonicae) and fear *Mu Meng* (Radix Et Ehizoma Paridis Tetraphyllae), *Di Yu* (Radix Sanguisorbae Officinalis), *Xiong Huang* (Realgar), *Qin Jiao* (Radix Gentianae Macrophyllae), and *Gui Jia* (Plastrum Testudinis).

Du Zhong (Cortex Eucommiae Ulmoidis) is averse to *She Tui* (Exuviae Serpentis) and *Yuan Shen* (Radix Scrophulariae Ningpoensis).

The envoys of *Bai Shi* (Semen Biotae Orientalis) are *Mu Li* (Concha Ostreae), *Gui Xin* (Cortex Rasus Cinnamomi Cassiae), and *Gua Zi* (Semen

173

Curcumeris). It is averse to *Ju Hua* (Flos Chrysanthemi Morifolii), *Yang Ti* (Radix Rumicis Japonici), various stones, and *Mian Qu* (Fermented Flour).

The envoy of *Gan Qi* (Lacca Sinica Exsiccata) is *Ban Xia* (Rhizoma Pinelliae Ternatae). It fears *Ji Zi* (Chicken Egg).

Man Jing Zi (Fructus Viticis) is averse to *Wu Tou* (Radix Aconiti) and *Shi Gao* (Gypsum).

The envoy of *Wu Jia Pi* (Cortex Radicis Acanthopanacis) is *Yuan Zhi* (Radix Polygalae Tenuifoliae). It fears *She Pi* (Exuviae Serpentis) and *Yuan Shen* (Radix Scrophulariae Ningpoensis).

Bai Mu (Lignum Biotae Orientalis) is averse to *Gan Qi* (Lacca Sinica Exsiccata).

The envoy of *Xin Yi* (Flos Magnoliae Liliflorae) is *Xiong Qiong* (Radix Ligustici Wallichii). It is averse to *Wu Shi Zhi* (the Five Halloysitums) and fears *Chang Pu* (Rhizoma Acori Graminei), *Pu Huang* (Pollen Typhae), *Huang Lian* (Rhizoma Coptidis Chinensis), *Shi Gao* (Gypsum), and *Huang Huan* (?).

Suan Zao Ren (Semen Zizyphi Spinosae) is averse to *Fang Ji* (Radix Stephaniae Tetrandrae).

The envoy of *Huai Zi* (Fructus Sophorae Japonicae) is *Jing Tian* (Herba Sedi Erythrosticti).

The envoy of *Mu Jing Shi* (Fructus Viticis Negundi) is *Fang Ji* (Radix Stephaniae Tetrandrae). It is averse to *Shi Gao* (Gypsum).

Woods: Middle Class

The envoy of *Hou Po* (Cortex Magnoliae Officinalis) is *Gan Jiang* (dry Rhizoma Jingiberis). It is averse to *Ze Xie* (Rhizoma Alismatis), *Han Shui Shi* (Calcareous Spar), and *Xiao Shi* (Niter).

The envoy of *Shan Zhu Yu* (Fructus Corni Officinalis) is *Liao Shi* (Fructus Polygoni Hydropiperis). It is averse to *Jie Geng* (Radix Platycodi Grandiflori), *Fang Feng* (Radix Ledebouriellae Divaricatae), and *Fang Ji* (Radix Stephaniae Tetrandrae).

The envoy of *Wu Zhu Yu* (Fructus Evodiae Rutecarpae) is *Liao Shi* (Fructus Polygoni Hydropiperis). It is averse to *Dan Shen* (Radix Salviae Miltiorrhizae), *Xiao Shi* (Niter), and *Bai Wu* (Kaolin or Chalk), and it fears *Zi Shi Ying* (Flouritum).

The envoy of *Qin Pi* (Cortex Fraxini) is *Da Ji* (Herba Seu Radix Cirsii Japonici). It is averse to *Zhu Yu* (Fructus Evodiae Rutecarpae).

Zhan Si (Cocoon of Monema Flavescens) resolves the toxins of *Lang Du* (Radix Stellerae Chamaejasmis).

Zhi Zi (Fructus Gardeniae Jasminoidis) resolves the toxins of *Zhi Zhu* (Flos Rhododendri Sublaneolati).

Qin Jiao (Pericarpium Zanthoxyli Bungeani) is averse to *Gua Lou* (Fructus Trichosanthis Kirlowii) and *Fang Kui* (Radix Peucedani Japonici), and it fears *Ci Huang* (Auripigmentum).

The envoys of *Sang Gen Bai Pi* (Cortex Radicis Mori Albi) are *Xu Duan* (Radix Dipsaci), *Gui Xin* (Cortex Rasus Cinnamomi Cassiae), and *Ma Zi* (Semen Cannabis Sativae).

Woods: Inferior Class

The envoy of *Huang Huan* (?) is *Yuan Wei* (Radix Et Rhizoma Iridis Tectori). It is averse to *Fu Ling* (Sclerotium Poriae Cocos) and *Fang Ji* (Radix Stephaniae Tetrandrae).

The envoy of *Shi Nan* (Folium Photiniae Serrulatae) is *Wu Jia Pi* (Cortex Radicis Acanthopanacis Garacilistyli).

The envoy of *Ba Dou* (Semen Crotonis Tiglii) is *Yuan Hua* (Flos Daphnes Genkwae). It is averse to *Rang Cao* (Folium Zingiberis Miogae), fears *Da Huang* (Radix Et Rhizoma Rhei), *Huang Lian* (Rhizoma Coptidis Chinensis), and *Li Lu* (Radix Et Rhizoma Veratri), and kills the toxins of *Ban Mao* (Mylabris).

The envoy of *Luan Hua* (Flos Koelreuteriae Paniculutae) is *Jue Ming* (Semen Cassiae Torae).

The envoy of *Shu Jiao* (Pericarpium Zanthoxyli Bungeani) is *Xing Ren* (Semen Pruni Armeniacae). It is averse to *Kuan Dong* (Flos Tussilaginis Farfarae).

The envoy of *Sou Shu* (Semen Deutziae Scabrae) is *Lou Lu* (Radix Echinponsis Seu Rhapontici).

The envoy of *Zao Jia* (Fructus Gleditschiae Chinensis) is *Bai Shi* (Semen Biotae Orientalis). It is averse to *Mai Men Dong* (Tuber Ophiopogonis Japonici) and fears *Kong Qing* (Azuritum), *Ren Shen* (Radix Panacis Ginseng), and *Ku Shen* (Radix Sophorae Flavescentis).

The envoys of *Lei Wan* (Fructificatio Polypori Mylittae) are *Li Shi* (Semen Iridis Pallasii) and *Hou Po* (Cortex Magnoliae Officinalis). It is averse to *Ge Gen* (Radix Puerariae).

Beasts: Superior Class

Long Gu (Os Draconis) will become better if it acquires *Ren Shen* (Radix Panacis Ginseng) and *Niu Huang* (Calculus Bovis). It fears *Shi Gao* (Gypsum).

Long Jiao (Cornu Draconis) fears *Gan Qi* (Lacca Sinica Exsiccata), *Shu Jiao* (Pericarpium Zanthoxyli Bungeani), and *Li Shi* (Gypsum Fibrosum).

The envoy of *Niu Huang* (Calculus Bovis) is *Ren Shen* (Radix Panacis Ginseng). It is averse to *Long Gu* (Os Draconis), *Di Huang* (Radix Rehmanniae), *Di Dan* (Meloe Coartatus), and *Fei Lian* (Stylopyga Conucina), and it fears *Niu Xi* (Radix Achyranthis Bidentatae).

Bai Jiao (Gelatinum Cornu Cervi) will become better if it acquires fire. It fears *Da Huang* (Radix Et Rhizoma Rhei).

E Jiao (Gelatinum Corii Asini) will become better if it acquires fire. It is averse to *Da Huang* (Radix Et Rhizoma Rhei).

Beasts: Middle Class

The envoy of *Xi Jiao* (Cornu Rhinocerotis) is *Song Zhi* (Resina Pini). It is averse to *Huan Jun* (Herba Phragmitis Communis) and *Lei Wan* (Fructificatio Polypori Mylittae).

The envoy of *Gu Yang Jiao* (Cornu Antelopis Saiga-tatarici) is *Tu Si Zi* (Semen Cuscutae Chinensis)

The envoy of *Lu Rong* (Cornu Parvum Cervi) is *Ma Bo* (Flos Cannabis Sativae at the time of pollenization).

The envoy of *Lu Jiao* (Cornu Cervi) is *Du Zhong* (Cortex Eucommiae Ulmoidis).

177

Beasts: Inferior Class

Mi Zhi (Adeps Elaphuri Davidiani) fears *Da Huang* (Radix Et Rhizoma Rhei).

The envoys of *Fu Yi* (Vesperugo Noctula) are *Xian Shi* (Semen Amaranthi) and *Yun Shi* (Semen Caesalpiniae Sepiariae).

Tian Shu Shi (Excrementum Verpertilionis Murini) is averse to *Bai Lian* (Radix Ampelopsis Japonicae) and *Bai Wei* (Radix Cynanchi Baiwei).

Insects, Worms and Fish: Superior Class

Mi La (Cera Alba) is averse to *Yuan Hua* (Flos Daphnes Genkwae) and *Qi Ge* (Mactra Quandrangularis).

Feng Zi (Larva Apis Ceranae) fears *Huang Qin* (Radix Scutellariae Baicalensis), *Shao Yao* (Radix Paeoniae Lactiflorae), and *Mu Li* (Concha Ostreae).

The envoy of *Mu Li* (Concha Ostreae) is *Bei Mu* (Bulbus Fritillariae). It will become better if it acquires *Gan Cao* (Radix Glycyrrhizae), *Niu Xi* (Radix Achyranthis Bidentatae), *Yuan Zhi* (Radix Polygalae Tenuifoliae), and *She Chuang Zi* (Fructus Cnidii Monnieri). It is averse to *Ma Huang* (Herba Ephedrae), *Wu Zhu Yu* (Fructus Evodiae Rutecarpae), *Xin Yi* (Flos Magnoliae Liliflorae), and *Sang Piao Xiao* (Ootheca Mantidis), and it fears *Xuan Fu Hua* (Flos Inulae).

The envoy of *Hai Ge* (Concha Cyclinae Sinensis) is *Shu Qi* (Folium Et Ramulus Dichroae Febrifugae). It fears *Gou Dan* (Fel Canis), *Gan Sui* (Radix Euphorbiae Kansui), and *Yuan Hua* (Flos Daphnis Genkwae).

Gui Jia (Plastrum Testudinis) is averse to *Sha Shen* (Radix Glehniae Littoralis) and *Fei Lian* (Stylopyga Conucina).

Insects, Worms and Fish: Middle Class

Wei Pi (Pellis Erinacei) will become better if it acquires wine. It fears *Jie Geng* (Radix Platycodi Grandiflori) and *Mai Men Dong* (Tuber Ophiopogonis Japonici).

Xi Yi (Eumeces Chinensis) is averse to *Liu Huang* (Sulphur), *Ban Mao* (Mylabris), and *Wu Yi* (Semen Praeparatus Ulmi Macrocarpae).

Lu Feng Fang (Nidus Vespae) is averse to *Gan Jiang* (dry Rhizoma Zingiberis), *Dan Shen* (Radix Salviae Miltiorrhizae), *Huang Qin* (Radix Scutellariae Baicalensis), *Shao Yao* (Radix Paeoniae Lactiflorae), and *Mu Li* (Concha Ostreae).

Zhe Chong (Eupolyphaga Seu Ophistoplatia) fears *Zao Jia* (Fructus Gleditschiae Chinensis) and *Chang Pu* (Rhizoma Acori Graminei).

The envoy of *Qi Cao* (Holotrichia Diomphalia) is *Fei Lian* (Stylopyga Conucina). It is averse to *Fu Zi* (Radix Lateralis Praeparatus Aconiti Carmichaeli).

Bie Jia (Carpax Amydae Sinensis) is averse to *Fan Shi* (Alumen).

Xie (Eriocheir Sinensis) kills the toxins of *Lang Dang* (Semen Scopoliae Japonicae) and *Qi* (Lacca Sinica Exsiccata).

The envoy of *Tuo Yu Jia* (Squama Alligatoris Sinensis) is *Shu Qi* (Folium Et Ramulus Dichroae Febrifugae). It fears *Gou Dan* (Fel Canis), *Gan Sui* (Radix Euphorbiae Kansui), and *Yuan Hua* (Flos Daphnis Genkwae).

Wu Zei Yu Gu (Os Sepiae Seu Sepiellae) is averse to *Bai Lian* (Radix Ampelopsis Japonicae) and *Bai Ji* (Rhizoma Bletillae Striatae).

Insects, Worms and Fish: Inferior Class

Qiang Lang (Geotrupes Laesistriatus) fears *Yang Jiao* (Cornu Caprae) and *Shi Gao* (Gypsum).

She Tui (Exuviae Serpentis) fears *Ci Shi* (Magnetitum) and wine.

The envoy of *Ban Mao* (Mylabris) is *Ma Dao* (Mactra Quandrangularis). It fears *Ba Dou* (Semen Crotonis Tiglii), *Dan Shen* (Radix Salviae Miltiorrhizae), and *Kong Qing* (Azuritum), and it is averse to *Fu Qing* (Azuritum).

Di Dan (Meloe Coartatus) is averse to *Gan Cao* (Radix Glycyrrhizae).

Fruits: Superior Class

Da Zao (Fructus Zizyphi Jujubae) kills the toxins of *Wu Tou* (Radix Aconiti).

Fruits: Inferior Class

Xing Ren (Semen Pruni Armeniacae) will become better if it acquires fire. It is averse to *Huang Qi* (Radix Astragali Membranacei), *Huang Qin* (Radix Scutellariae Baicalensis), and *Ge Gen* (Radix Puerariae), resolves the toxins of *Xi Hu Fen* (Carbonate of Lead), and fears *Rang Cao* (Folium Zingiberis Miogae).

Vegetables: Superior Class

The envoy of *Dong Kui Zi* (Semen Abutilonis Seu Malvae) is *Huang Qin* (Radix Scutellariae Baicalensis).

Cong Shi (Semen Allii Fistulosi) resolves the toxins of *Li Lu* (Radix Et Rhizoma Veratri).

Cereals: Superior Class

Ma Fen (Flos Cannabis Sativae) and *Ma Zi* (Semen Cannabis Sativae) fear *Mu Li* (Concha Ostreae) and *Bai Wei* (Radix Cynanchi Baiwei) and are averse to *Fu Ling* (Sclerotium Poriae Cocos).

Cereals: Middle Class

Da Dou (Semen Glycinis Hispidae) and *Huang Juan* (Semen Germinatus Glycinis Hispidae) are averse to *Wu Shen* (the Five *Shen, i.e.,* Radix Panacis Ginseng, Radix Salviae Miltiorrhizae, Radix Glehniae Littoralis, Radix Scrophulariae Ningpoensis, and Radix Pseustellariae Heterophyllae) and *Long Dan* (Radix Gentianae Scabrae). They will become better if they acquire *Qian Hu* (Radix Peucedani), *Wu Hui* (Radix Aconiti), *Xing Ren* (Semen Pruni Armeniacae), and *Mu Li* (Concha Ostreae). They kill the toxins of *Wu Tou* (Radix Aconiti).

The envoy of *Da Mai* (Semen Hordei Vulgaris) is *Mi* (Mel).

[Here ends the section on Cereals: Middle Class.]

The above 231 medicinals have restrainers and envoys, while others do not.

On the day, Beginning of Winter, *Ju* (Chrysanthemum) and *Juan Bai* (Selaginella Tamariscina) first begin to grow. Then 10 materials, including

181

Yang Qi Shi (Actinolitum) and *Sang Piao Xiao* (Ootheca Mantidis), come into use as envoys.[408] [This season] governs the growth of 200 herbs.[409]

On the day, Beginning of Spring, *Mu Lan* (Magnolia Liliflora) and *She Gan* (Belamcanda Chinensis) first begin to grow. *Chai Hu* (Radix Bupleuri) and *Ban Xia* (Rhizoma Pinelliae Ternatae) come into use as envoys.[408] [This season] governs headache[409] and 45 joints.

On the day, Beginning of Summer, *Fei Lian* (Stylopyga Conucina) first begins to grow. *Ren Shen* (Radix Panacis Ginseng) and *Fu Ling* (Sclerotium Poriae Cocos) come into use as envoys.[408] [This season] governs abdominal inside and seven joints.[409] [These medicinals] protect the spirit and safeguard the center.

On the day, Summer Solstice, *Shi Shou* (Iris Pallasium) and *Zhu Yu* (Evodia Rutecarpa) first begin to grow. *Mu Li* (Concha Ostreae) and *Wu Hui* (Radix Aconiti) come into use as envoys.[408] [This season] governs the four limbs and 32 joints.[409]

On the day, Beginning of Autumn, *Bai Zhi* (Angelica Dahurica) and *Fang Feng* (Ledebouriella Divaricata) first begin to grow.[410] *Xi Xin* (Herba Asari Cum Radice) and *Shu Qi* (Folium Et Ramulus Dichroae Febrifugae) come

---

[408] Regarding this sentence, there is another interpretation, which says that, after the Beginning of Winter, *Yang Qi Shi* (Actinolitum) has *Sang Piao Xiao* (Ootheca Mantidis) as its envoy. The next four passages each contain a similar statement which may be understood in this alternative way.

[409] This sentence may be translated in a number of other ways. One has it that *Yang Qi Shi* (Actinolitum), etc. govern (or treat) 200 (joints) and weeds begin to grow. The next passages each contain a similar statement which may also be interpreted in this way.

[410] The words "begin to grow" mean "ripening" or "beginning to bear fruit."

into use as envoys.[408] [This season] governs the chest, (upper) back, and 24 joints.[409, 411]

---

[411] All five of the above passages are about the seasonal law concerning the use of medicinals. They are from the *Yao Dui (Questions & Answers About Medicinals)* supposedly written by Tong Jun. Tong Jun was said to be one of the ministers of the Yellow Emperor. However, most scholars in the past have thought these passages to be derived from the *Ben Cao Jing*.

Addendum

Gua Lou (Trichosanthes Kirlowium) has leaves like those of [water] melon which grow by twos, opposite to one another. It is blackish green-blue. It crawls up, bearing flowers in the sixth month and yielding fruit in the seventh month which look like a slice of melon.

Yan Mai (Bromus Japonicus) grows in the wilderness and forest. Its stalk looks like that of wheat but weaker. Its seed looks like barley but is thinner. It is also seen in other places.

Ji (Capsella Bursa-pastoris) is sweet. People pick its leaves as a food after they are seasoned. They can make soup which is also good.

Du Heng (Asarum Forbesium) is acrid and can be used to fumigate the body and clothes.

Shi Yun (Molsa Chinensis) is also named *Zhe Lie* (Terrible Biting). Its other name is *Gui Hui* (Inquisitive Beak).

Fei Li (Blatta Orientalis) is an insect.

Guan Gu (Os Ciconiae Ciconiae) is sweet. It is nontoxic, treating demonic and worm influx and the five cadavers[412] causing disease in the heart and abdomen.

In spring, *Yuan Qing* (Daphnes Genkwae) offers its flower to be taken. For that reason, it is called *Yuan Qing* (Evergreen Daphne). In autumn,

---

[412] The five cadavers include flying cadaver (*fei shi*), fleeing cadaver (*dun shi*), cold cadaver (*han shi*), bereaved cadaver (*sang shi*), and cadaverous influx (*shu zhu*). This is a general term for fatal infectious disease.

[Daphnes Genkwae] offers *Di Dan* (Meloe Coartatus).[413] [Meloe Coartatus,] which has a black head and red tail, is toxic, mainly treats worm toxins and wind influx. In autumn, people take *Ge Hua* (Flos Puerariae). Therefore, [Flos Puerariae] is called *Ge Shang Ting Zhang* (Over-pavilion Vine).

That which branches from the root of mulberry and emerges from earth is named *Fu She* (Lying Snake). It treats heart pain. *Sang Gen Bai Pi* (Cortex Radicis Mori Albi) is the white bark of the mulberry root. It is usually collected in the fourth month but may be collected any time [throughout the year]. That [part of the root] which is seen above the earth is called *Ma Ling* (Horse Collar). Do not collect it because its toxins may kill people.

He Huan (Albizzia Julibrissinis) grows in Yu Zhou[414] in rivers and valleys. The tree looks like *Gou Gu Shu* (Ilex Cornuta).[415]

Shi Fei (Calcitum) is also called *Shi Gan* (Stone Liver). Shiny black with red striations, it looks like an upside-down liver. Once put in water, it becomes dry.[416] It mainly boosts the qi and brightens the eyes. It is produced in the water.

Shi Pi (Limonitum)[417] is also called *Wei Shi* (Stone Stomach) and *Shen Shi* (Stone Kidney). It has a red texture. It mainly treats cold and heat in the stomach.

---

[413] This sentence implies that *Di Dan* (Meloe Coartatus) is the root of Daphnes. Actually, it is an insect growing *around* the root of Daphnes. This insect is then caught and dried in autumn.

[414] Its precincts were roughly those of present-day Henan Province.

[415] These two kinds of tree do not resemble one another.

[416] According to descriptions in other reliable works, like the *Zhong Guo Yi Xue Da Ci Dian (A Dictionary of Chinese Medicine)*, the meaning of this sentence is, "Taken out of water, it immediately becomes dry."

[417] This is a slightly yellow stone, bean-shaped with red striations.

Qing Shi Zhi (Halloysitum Indicum) is sour and balanced. It is nontoxic, mainly nourishing the qi of the liver and gallbladder. *Chi Shi Zhi* (Halloysitum Rubrum) is sour. It is nontoxic, nourishing the heart qi. *Huang Shi Zhi* (Hallyositum Aureum) is balanced of flavor. It is nontoxic, mainly nourishing the spleen qi. *Bai Shi Zhi* (Hallyositum Album) is sweet. It is nontoxic, mainly nourishing the lung qi. *Hei Shi Zhi* (Hallyositum Atrum) is sweet. It is nontoxic, mainly nourishing the kidney qi, fortifying yin and yang, and [treating] intestinal erosion diarrhea and dysentery.

Ceng Qing (Azuritum) is produced in the famous mountains of Shu Prefecture where copper is produced. *Ceng Qing* (Azuritum) is produced on the south side of these mountains. [The color] green-blue[418] is the essence of copper and [therefore] is able to transform into golden and copper.

Lu Zhi (Adeps Cervi) may make one impotent if one is in [constant] contact with it.

Yuan (Milvus Korchun) keeps away ill matters. It grows in Huai Nan.[419]

Ku Shen (Radix Sophorae Flavescentis) is also named *Shui Huai* (Water Scholartree).

Ren Dong (Ramus Lonicerae Japonicae) is sweet. Prolonged taking may make the body light.

Ling Ruo (Campsis Grandiflora) grows in low, damp lands and in water. It blooms in the seventh and eighth months. Its flower is purple and it looks like the golden flower of *Zi Cao* (Lithospermum Seu Arnebia). It may dye cloth. After being boiled, it may be used to wash the hair which will turn black in no time.

---

[418] In the name *Ceng Qing*, the word *qing* means green-blue.

[419] *I.e.*, south of the Huai River

Xuan (Hemerocallis Fulva) is also called *Wang Yu* (Worry-freeing Weed), *Yi Nan* (Good for Men) and *Qi Nu* (Woman Discrimination).

When the tiger roars, wind will blow. When the dragon booms, clouds will gather. Magnetitum (*Ci*) can attract needles, and Succinum (*Hu*) can pick up mustard seeds. When *Qi* (Lacca Sinica Exsiccata) meets with *Xie* (Eriocheir Sinensis), it is dispersed. When *Ma* (Semen Cannabis Sativae) meets with *Qi* (Lacca Sinica Exsiccata),[420] it will cause ejection. If *Gui* (Cortex Cinnamomi Cassiae) meets with *Cong* (Bulbus Allii Fistulosi), it will become soft. If the (lacquer) tree touches Cassia, it will wither.[421] *Rong Yan* (Alkali) exists in the form of overlying eggs, while *Ta Dan* (Fel Lutrae Lutrae) is divided when it is put in the cup. [All this shows that things] are interrelated although their qi are different. They act upon each other.

[420] *Qi* (Lacca Sinica Exsiccata) is toxic. If one is poisoned by it, *Xie* (Eriocheir Sinensis) may resolve it. One action of *Ma* (Semen Cannabis Sativae) is downbearing to treat, for example, constipation and scanty urine. If it meets with *Xie* (Eriocheir Sinensis), its downbearing action will become reversed. Then it will upbear.

[421] The translator has failed to find an authentic explanation for the preceding two sentences.

General Index

A

A Barefoot Doctor's Manual, vi
A Classic & Historic [Work]: A Materia Medica for Emergencies, iv
abscesses, flat, 6-10, 12, 16, 21, 37, 38, 45, 48, 55, 57, 64, 66, 67, 73, 77, 78, 82, 86, 88, 103, 106, 108, 131, 135
abdomen, enlarged xv, 35, 63, 69-71, 105-107, 113
abdomen, hardness and pain in, 13
abdomen, severe pain in the heart and, 26
abdomen, water qi in the, 29
abdominal heat pain, 48
abdominal mounting qi, 103
abdominal pain, xiii, xv, 3, 10, 33, 34, 45, 49, 63, 65, 75, 80, 88, 102-105, 114, 116, 120, 135, 141
abdominal pain, cute xiii
abdominal rumbling, 65
abortion, 3, 26, 82, 101, 105, 126, 129, 132, 135
abortion, induces, 3, 26, 105, 129, 132, 135
abscesses and swelling, 130
aching pain everywhere, xiii
aging, slow, 23, 26, 27, 29, 32-36, 47, 83, 84, 89, 91, 93, 95, 100, 103, 115, 139, 140, 142
allergic skin rashes, 30
anus, splitting of the 37
anus, swollen tubercles or pustulation around the, 37
appendicitis, 145
appetite, no, xvi
arched-back rigidity, xv
arthritis, rheumatic, 87
assistants, iii, ix-xi

B

back, pain and rigidity of the upper and lower, 56
back, rigidity of in children, 90
baldness, 10, 64, 79, 80, 113
bandit wind, 14, 59, 73, 78, 124
belching, 66
Ben Cao Gang Mu, iv, vii, 116
bend or stretch, inability to, 26, 59
beng lou, 10
bladder, heat bound in the, 28
bleeding wounds, 36
blindness, xvi, 3, 11, 36, 43, 77, 118, 120, 130, 140
blindness, clear-eye, 3, 36, 77, 118, 120
blindness, night, 130
blood amassment in the lower burner, 87
blood block, xvi, 6, 16, 42, 45, 48, 58, 60, 69, 72, 101, 114, 115, 123, 126, 131, 145
blood diseases, 102
blood, dribbling of, from the vagina, 10
blood ejection, xiii, xv, 67, 111, 114, 119, 120, 139, 142, 146
blood, hacking of, 49, 52
blood impediment, 20, 49, 83, 97, 99
blood, malign, 10, 43, 49, 79, 120, 121, 124, 131, 149
blood, precipitation of, 6, 9
blood stasis, xiv, 9, 21, 29, 35, 36, 54, 60, 66-69, 99, 113, 121, 123, 131, 145, 149
blood stasis in the five viscera, 29
bone damage, xvi
bone pain, 120
bones, broken, xvi, 46
bones, heat in the, 31
bones, steaming, 47, 55, 67, 93, 125, 141
brain, shaking, 26
bravery and undauntedness, 18
breast milk stoppage, 41, 43
breath, bad, 142
breath, inability to catch one's, 13, 112

breathing, faint, 112
breathing, inhibited, xv, 88
breathing, rough, 24
burns, 13, 26, 35, 48, 57, 77, 78, 92, 133

C

cadavers, five, 183
canthi, injured, 34, 107, 123
canthi, ulcered 14
Cao Yuan-yu, v
center, damaged, 20-22, 25, 26, 42, 46,
    101, 109, 114, 116, 120, 121, 123,
    147, 149
chest and rib-side pain, 29, 65, 84
chest binding, 65, 98, 143
chest, bound heat in the, 35
chest, bound phlegm in the, 77
chest, enduring cold in the, 5
chest fullness, xvi, 34, 50, 51, 65, 69, 74
chest fullness and glomus, xvi
choleraic disease, 31, 73, 87, 96
Cinnabar, 2, 17, 82, 100, 116, 122, 123,
    132, 155, 159, 167
clove toxins, 34
cold damage, xv, 17, 28, 37, 46, 51, 53,
    69, 71, 73, 75, 77, 87, 96, 97, 100,
    103-108, 115, 117, 119, 142, 143
collapse, 31, 113, 119, 158
collapse, sudden, 112
concretions and conglomerations, xvi,
    3, 6, 15, 16, 26, 31, 43, 44, 47, 54,
    55, 69, 73, 74, 75, 78, 79, 88, 94, 98,
    101, 102, 106, 113, 117, 125, 126,
    127, 132, 136
consciousness, loss of, xi, 31, 60, 108,
    119
consciousness, sudden loss of, xi, 60
constipation, 74, 108, 143, 186
corpse, hidden, 15, 19, 133, 134
cough, xv, xvi, 5, 6, 9, 15, 18, 20, 21,
    24, 26, 28, 39, 41, 43, 45-48, 50-53,
    59, 61, 62, 65, 69-76, 81, 82, 85-88,
    96-101, 104, 106, 109, 112, 115, 116,

124, 125, 133, 140, 143, 145
cough, enduring, 81, 109, 125
cough, lung heat, 48
cough, phlegm 69
cough, taxation, 20
cough with ejection of pus, blood, 59
crippling wilt, 59, 73

D

damp impediment, 5, 19, 21-23, 25, 26,
    29, 33, 38-39, 47, 50, 59, 61, 63, 66,
    72-73, 81, 83, 87, 89, 92, 95, 98-99,
    106-107, 118, 125, 130, 137, 149
Dao Guang, vi
dead blood, 96
deafness, xvi, 3, 11, 18, 68, 98, 105,
    115, 133
deafness, kidney vacuity, 11
death, premature, 27
defecation, abnormal xvi
delirium, 119, 134
delivery, difficult 26, 52, 61, 125, 134
delivery, hasten, 44, 120, 126, 148
demonic influx, xiii, xv, xvi, 14, 33, 35,
    38, 45, 64, 71, 74, 76, 82, 84, 104,
    112, 129, 130, 132-135, 145
demonology, vii, 2
derangement, xiii, 2
dermatoses, 95
diarrhea, xv, 3, 5, 6, 9, 10, 14, 15, 19,
    24, 28, 29, 31, 35, 37, 42, 47-51, 62,
    70, 72, 73, 87, 91, 93, 96, 98, 101,
    105, 112, 114, 120, 142, 151, 185
diarrhea, cold, 10, 120
disease, enduring, 24
diseases, sudden, 27
dizziness, 4, 22, 23, 44, 58, 75, 83, 121
dizziness, wind head, 44
dizziness, wind phlegm, 83
dog bite, rabid 38
dreams, ghost, 31, 113, 119, 120
dribbling block, 18, 33
drinker's nose, 96, 100, 114

L

lacquer sores, 99, 126
lactation, difficult, 5, 22, 43, 46, 53, 121, 123
lactation, promotes, 9, 10, 13, 38, 116, 143
lai disease, 16, 37, 96
lai, red, 100
lai, white, 100
Large Dictionary of Chinese Medicinals, vi
leg, sores on the lower, 15
legs, heaviness and aching pain in the lower, 75
legs, sores on the lower, 15
lice on the skin, 2
limb distention, 59
limb fullness, 60
limb joints, pain in the, 11, 20, 48, 80
limbs, aching pain in the, 63, 83, 92, 114
limbs, cold, 11, 23, 73, 141
limbs, heaviness of the, xiii, 125, 138
limbs, heaviness and weakness of the, 125
limbs, hypertonicity of the, 26, 71
limbs, insensitivity of the, 20, 96
limbs, obstinate impediment of the, 21
limbs, puffy swelling of the, 52, 70
limbs, face, and eyes, puffy swelling of the, 70
limbs, reversal cold of the, 11, 23, 73
limpness, 103
lips and mouth, dryness of the, 41
listlessness, 46
lockjaw, 64, 83, 132
longevity, extreme, x
lower burner, blood amassment in the, 87
lumbago, 20, 43, 46, 63, 88, 90, 114, 123, 125
lumbus, pain in the, 26, 29, 32, 43, 63, 89, 115, 122-123, 126, 139

lumbus and knees, pain in the, 32, 43, 89, 122, 141
lung abscesses, 65
lung fire, 13, 24, 41, 48, 92, 93
lung heat rapid panting, 60
lung wilting, 29, 41, 43, 52, 62
lung wilting ejection of blood, 41
lying beam, 76

M

macular eruption, 55
madness, 15, 37, 81, 112, 123, 130-132
malaria, mother of 74
malaria, warm, xv, 28, 39, 51, 59, 60, 71, 74, 78, 79, 83, 105, 113, 117, 132
mania, 12, 34, 79, 97, 108, 111, 112, 119, 120, 134
mania, heat, 34
manic vexation, 14
masses in the rib-side region, xiii
medicinals, cold, ii, xiii
medicinals, hot, ii, xiii, 73
medicinals, inferior class, ix, x, 153
medicinals, medium class, x
medicinals, superior class, ix, 153
medicinals, toxic, xii-xiv
medicinals, wound, xiii
Medicine in China: A History of Pharmaceutics, iii, vi, vii
memory, 21, 32, 34, 57, 123
menses, desiccated 41
menstrual block, 15, 68, 74, 124, 131, 133
menstruation, postmenopausal recommencement of, 48
mental disorders, 7, 27, 106
mental-neurological problems, xi
miasmic evils, 27
mind, confused, 60
ministers, iii, ix-xi, 182
miscarriage, threatened, 105
moles and polyps, black, 16
mounting conglomeration, 27, 28, 49,

Medicinal Index in Latin

Medicinal Index in Pin Yin

OTHER BOOKS ON CHINESE MEDICINE AVAILABLE FROM:
BLUE POPPY ENTERPRISES, INC.
Colorado: 1990 North 57th Court, Unit A, Boulder, CO 80301
For ordering 1-800-487-9296 PH. 303-447-8372 FAX 303-245-8362
California: 1725 Monrovia Ave. Unit A4, Costa Mesa, CA 92627
For ordering 1-800-293-6697 PH. 949-270-6511 FAX 949-335-7110
Email: info@bluepoppy.com Website: www.bluepoppy.com

ACUPOINT POCKET REFERENCE
by Bob Flaws
ISBN 0-936185-93-7
ISBN 978-0-936185-93-4

ACUPUNCTURE, CHINESE MEDICINE & HEALTHY
WEIGHT LOSS   Revised Edition
by Juliette Aiyana, L. Ac.
ISBN 1-891845-61-6
ISBN 978-1-891845-61-1

ACUPUNCTURE & IVF
by Lifang Liang
ISBN 0-891845-24-1
ISBN 978-0-891845-24-6

ACUPUNCTURE FOR STROKE REHABILITATION
Three Decades of Information from China
by Hoy Ping Yee Chan, et al.
ISBN 1-891845-35-7
ISBN 978-1-891845-35-2

ACUPUNCTURE PHYSICAL MEDICINE: An
Acupuncture Touchpoint Approach to the Treatment
of Chronic Pain, Fatigue, and Stress Disorders
by Mark Seem
ISBN 1-891845-13-6
ISBN 978-1-891845-13-0

AGING & BLOOD STASIS: A New Approach to TCM
Geriatrics
by Yan De-xin
ISBN 0-936185-63-6
ISBN 978-0-936185-63-7

AN ACUPUNCTURISTS GUIDE TO MEDICAL RED
FLAGS & REFERRALS
by Dr. David Anzaldua, MD
ISBN 1-891845-54-3
ISBN 978-1-891845-54-3

BETTER BREAST HEALTH NATURALLY with
CHINESE MEDICINE
by Honora Lee Wolfe & Bob Flaws
ISBN 0-936185-90-2
ISBN 978-0-936185-90-3

BIOMEDICINE: A TEXTBOOK FOR PRACTITIONERS
OF ACUPUNCTURE AND ORIENTAL MEDICINE
by Bruce H. Robinson, MD Second Edition
ISBN 1-891845-62-4
ISBN 978-1-891845-62-8

THE BOOK OF JOOK: Chinese Medicinal Porridges
by Bob Flaws
ISBN 0-936185-60-6
ISBN 978-0-936185-60-0

CHANNEL DIVERGENCES Deeper Pathways of the
Web
by Miki Shima and Charles Chase
ISBN 1-891845-15-2
ISBN 978-1-891845-15-4

CHINESE MEDICAL OBSTETRICS
by Bob Flaws
ISBN 1-891845-30-6
ISBN 978-1-891845-30-7

CHINESE MEDICAL PALM IS TRY: Your Health in
Your Hand
by Zong Xiao-fan & Gary Liscum
ISBN 0-936185-64-3
ISBN 978-0-936185-64-4

CHINESE MEDICAL PSYCHIATRY: A Textbook and
Clinical Manual
by Bob Flaws and James Lake, MD
ISBN 1-845891-17-9
ISBN 978-1-845891-17-8

CHINESE MEDICINAL TEAS: Simple, Proven, Folk
Formulas for Common Diseases & Promoting Health
by Zong Xiao-fan & Gary Lis cum
ISBN 0-936185-76-7
ISBN 978-0-936185-76-7

CHINESE MEDICINAL WINES & ELIXIRS
by Bob Flaws Revised Edition
ISBN 0-936185-58-9
ISBN 978-0-936185-58-3

CHINESE PEDIATRIC MASSAGE THERAPY: A
Parent's & Practitioner's Guide to the Prevention &
Treatment of Childhood Illness
by Fan Ya-li
ISBN 0-936185-54-6
ISBN 978-0-936185-54-5

CHINESE SCALP ACUPUNCTURE
by Jason Jishun Hao & Linda Lingzhi Hao
ISBN 1-891845-60-8
ISBN 978-1-891845-60-4

CHINESE SELF-MASSAGE THERAPY: The Easy
Way to Health
by Fan Ya-li
ISBN 0-936185-74-0
ISBN 978-0-936185-74-3

THE CLASSIC OF DIFFICULTIES: A Translation of
the Nan Jing
translation by Bob Flaws
ISBN 1-891845-07-1
ISBN 978-1-891845-07-9

A CLINICIAN'S GUIDE TO USING GRANULE
EXTRACTS
by Eric Brand
ISBN 1-891845-51-9
ISBN 978-1-891845-51-2

A COMPENDIUM OF CHINESE MEDICAL MEN-
STRUAL DISEASES
by Bob Flaws
ISBN 1-891845-31-4
ISBN 978-1-891845-31-4

CONCISE CHINESE MATERIA MEDICA
by Eric Brand and Nigel Wiseman
ISBN 0-912111-82-8
ISBN 978-0-912111-82-7

CONTEMPORARY GYNECOLOGY: An Integrated
Chinese-Western Approach
by Lifang Liang
ISBN 1-891845-50-0
ISBN 978-1-891845-50-5

CONTROLLING DIABETES NATURALLY WITH
CHINESE MEDICINE
by Lynn Kuchinski
ISBN 0-936185-06-3
ISBN 978-0-936185-06-2

CURING ARTHRITIS NATURALLY WITH CHINESE
MEDICINE
by Douglas Frank & Bob Flaws
ISBN 0-936185-87-2
ISBN 978-0-936185-87-3

CURING DEPRESSION NATURALLY WITH
CHINESE MEDICINE
by Rosa Schnyer & Bob Flaws
ISBN 0-936185-94-5
ISBN 978-0-936185-94-1

CURING FIBROMYALGIA NATURALLY WITH
CHINESE MEDICINE
by Bob Flaws
ISBN 1-891845-09-8
ISBN 978-1-891845-09-3

CURING HAY FEVER NATURALLY WITH CHINESE
MEDICINE
by Bob Flaws
ISBN 0-936185-91-0
ISBN 978-0-936185-91-0

CURING HEADACHES NATURALLY WITH
CHINESE MEDICINE
by Bob Flaws
ISBN 0-936185-95-3
ISBN 978-0-936185-95-8

CURING IBS NATURALLY WITH CHINESE
MEDICINE
by Jane Bean Oberski
ISBN 1-891845-11-X
ISBN 978-1-891845-11-6

CURING INSOMNIA NATURALLY WITH CHINESE
MEDICINE
by Bob Flaws
ISBN 0-936185-86-4
ISBN 978-0-936185-86-6

CURING PMS NATURALLY WITH CHINESE
MEDICINE
by Bob Flaws
ISBN 0-936185-85-6
ISBN 978-0-936185-85-9

DISEASES OF THE KIDNEY & BLADDER
by Hoy Ping Yee Chan, et al.
ISBN 1-891845-37-3
ISBN 978-1-891845-35-6

THE DIVINE FARMER'S MATERIA MEDICA: A
Translation of the Shen Nong Ben Cao
translation by Yang Shouz-zhong
ISBN 0-936185-96-1
ISBN 978-0-936185-96-5

DUI YAO: THE ART OF COMBINING CHINESE
HERBAL MEDICINALS
by Philippe Sionneau
ISBN 0-936185-81-3
ISBN 978-0-936185-81-1

ENDOMETRIOSIS, INFERTILITY AND TRADITIONAL
CHINESE MEDICINE: A Layperson's Guide
by Bob Flaws
ISBN 0-936185-14-7
ISBN 978-0-936185-14-9

THE ESSENCE OF LIU FENG-WU'S GYNECOLOGY
by Liu Feng-wu, translated by Yang Shou-zhong
ISBN 0-936185-88-0
ISBN 978-0-936185-88-0

EXTRA TREATISES BASED ON INVESTIGATION &
INQUIRY: A Translation of Zhu Dan-xi's Ge Zhi Yu Lun
translation by Yang Shou-zhong
ISBN 0-936185-53-8
ISBN 978-0-936185-53-8

FIRE IN THE VALLEY: TCM Diagnosis & Treatment of
Vaginal Diseases
by Bob Flaws
ISBN 0-936185-25-2
ISBN 978-0-936185-25-5

FULFILLING THE ESSENCE:
A Handbook of Traditional & Contemporary
Treatments for Female Infertility
by Bob Flaws
ISBN 0-936185-48-1
ISBN 978-0-936185-48-4

FU QING-ZHU'S GYNECOLOGY
trans. by Yang Shou-zhong and Liu Da-wei
ISBN 0-936185-35-X
ISBN 978-0-936185-35-4

GOLDEN NEEDLE WANG LE-TING: A 20th Century
Master's Approach to Acupuncture
by Yu Hui-chan and Han Fu-ru, trans. by Shuai Xue-
zhong
ISBN 0-936185-78-3
ISBN 978-0-936185-78-1

A HANDBOOK OF CHINESE HEMATOLOGY
by Simon Becker
ISBN 1-891845-16-0
ISBN 978-1-891845-16-1

A HANDBOOK OF TCM PATTERNS & THEIR
TREATMENTS
Second Edition
by Bob Flaws & Daniel Finney
ISBN 0-936185-70-8
ISBN 978-0-936185-70-5

A HANDBOOK OF TRADITIONAL CHINESE
DERMATOLOGY
by Liang Jian-hui, trans. by Zhang Ting-liang
& Bob Flaws
ISBN 0-936185-46-5
ISBN 978-0-936185-46-0

A HANDBOOK OF TRADITIONAL CHINESE
GYNECOLOGY
by Zhejiang College of TCM, trans. by Zhang Ting-
liang & Bob Flaws
ISBN 0-936185-06-6 (4th edit.)
ISBN 978-0-936185-06-4

A HANDBOOK of TCM PEDIATRICS
by Bob Flaws
ISBN 0-936185-72-4
ISBN 978-0-936185-72-9

THE HEART & ESSENCE OF DAN-XI'S METHODS OF TREATMENT
by Xu Dan-xi, trans. by Yang Shou-zhong
ISBN 0-926185-50-3
ISBN 978-0-936185-50-7

HERB TOXICITIES & DRUG INTERACTIONS: A Formula Approach
by Fred Jennes with Bob Flaws
ISBN 1-891845-26-8
ISBN 978-1-891845-26-0

IMPERIAL SECRETS OF HEALTH & LONGEVITY
by Bob Flaws
ISBN 0-936185-51-1
ISBN 978-0-936185-51-4

INSIGHTS OF A SENIOR ACUPUNCTURIST
by Miriam Lee
ISBN 0-936185-33-3
ISBN 978-0-936185-33-0

INTEGRATED PHARMACOLOGY: Combining Modern Pharmacology with Chinese Medicine
by Dr. Greg Sperber with Bob Flaws
ISBN 1-891845-41-1
ISBN 978-0-936185-41-3

INTRODUCTION TO THE USE OF PROCESSED CHINESE MEDICINALS
by Philippe Sionneau
ISBN 0-936185-62-7
ISBN 978-0-936185-62-0

KEEPING YOUR CHILD HEALTHY WITH CHINESE MEDICINE
by Bob Flaws
ISBN 0-936185-71-6
ISBN 978-0-936185-71-2

THE LAKESIDE MASTER'S STUDY OF THE PULSE
by Li Shi-zhen, trans. by Bob Flaws
ISBN 1-891845-01-2
ISBN 978-1-891845-01-7

MANAGING MENOPAUSE NATURALLY WITH CHINESE MEDICINE
by Honora Lee Wolfe
ISBN 0-936185-98-8
ISBN 978-0-936185-98-9

MASTER HUA'S CLASSIC OF THE CENTRAL VISCERA
by Hua Tuo, trans. by Yang Shou-zhong
ISBN 0-936185-43-0
ISBN 978-0-936185-43-9

THE MEDICAL I CHING: Oracle of the Healer Within
by Miki Shima
ISBN 0-936185-38-4
ISBN 978-0-936185-38-5

MENOPAIUSE & CHINESE MEDICINE
by Bob Flaws
ISBN 1-891845-40-3
ISBN 978-1-891845-40-6

MOXIBUSTION: A MODERN CLINICAL HANDBOOK
by Lorraine Wilcox
ISBN 1-891845-49-7
ISBN 978-1-891845-49-9

MOXIBUSTION: THE POWER OF MUGWORT FIRE
by Lorraine Wilcox
ISBN 1-891845-46-2
ISBN 978-1-891845-46-8

A NEW AMERICAN ACUPUNTURE By Mark Seem
ISBN 0-936185-44-9
ISBN 978-0-936185-44-6

PLAYING THE GAME: A Step-by-Step Approach to Accepting Insurance as an Acupuncturist
by Greg Sperber & Tiffany Anderson-Hefner
ISBN 3-131416-11-7
ISBN 978-3-131416-11-7

POCKET ATLAS OF CHINESE MEDICINE
Edited by Marne and Kevin Ergil
ISBN 1-891-845-59-4
ISBN 978-1-891845-59-8

POINTS FOR PROFIT: The Essential Guide to Practice Success for Acupuncturists   5th Fully Edited Edition
by Honora Wolfe with Marilyn Allen
ISBN 1-891845-25-X
ISBN 978-1-891845-25-3

PRINCIPLES OF CHINESE MEDICAL ANDROLOGY: An Integrated Approach to Male Reproductive and Urological Health by Bob Damone
ISBN 1-891845-45-4
ISBN 978-1-891845-45-1

PRINCE WEN HUI's COOK: Chinese Dietary Therapy
By Bob Flaws & Honora Wolfe
ISBN 0-912111-05-4
ISBN 978-0-912111-05-6

THE PULSE CLASSIC: A Translation of the Mai Jing
by Wang Shu-he, trans. by Yang Shou-zhong
ISBN 0-936185-75-9
ISBN 978-0-936185-75-0

THE SECRET OF CHINESE PULSE DIAGNOSIS
by Bob Flaws
ISBN 0-936185-67-8
ISBN 978-0-936185-67-5

SECRET SHAOLIN FORMULAS FOR THE TREATMENT OF EXTERNAL INJURY
by De Chan, trans. by Zhang Ting-liang & Bob Flaws
ISBN 0-936185-08-2
ISBN 978-0-936185-08-8

STATEMENTS OF FACT IN TRADITIONAL CHINESE MEDICINE   Revised & Expanded
by Bob Flaws
ISBN 0-936185-52-X
ISBN 978-0-936185-52-1

STICKING TO THE POINT: A Step-by-Step Approach to TCM Acupuncture Therapy   2 Condensed Books
by Bob Flaws & Honora Wolfe
ISBN 1-891845-47-0
ISBN 978-1-891845-47-5

A STUDY OF DAOIST ACUPUNCTURE
by Liu Zheng-cai
ISBN 1-891845-08-X
ISBN 978-1-891845-08-6

THE SUCCESSFUL CHINESE HERBALIST
by Bob Flaws and Honora Lee Wolfe
ISBN 1-891845-29-2
ISBN 978-1-891845-29-1

THE SYSTEMATIC CLASSIC OF ACUPUNCTURE & MOXIBUSTION: A translation of the Jia Yi Jing
by Huang-fu Mi, trans. by Yang Shou-zhong & Charles Chace
ISBN 0-936185-29-5
ISBN 978-0-936185-29-3

THE TAO OF HEALTHY EATING: DIETARY WISDOM ACCORDING TO CHINESE MEDICINE
by Bob Flaws Second Edition
ISBN 0-936185-92-9
ISBN 978-0-936185-92-7

TEACH YOURSELF TO READ MODERN MEDICAL
CHINESE
by Bob Flaws
ISBN 0-936185-99-6
ISBN 978-0-936185-99-6

TEST PREP WORKBOOK FOR BASIC TCM THEORY
by Zhong Bai-song
ISBN 1-891845-43-8
ISBN 978-1-891845-43-7

TEST PREP WORKBOOK FOR THE NCCAOM
BIOMEDICINE MODULE: Exam Preparation &
Study Guide
by Zhong Bai-song
ISBN 1-891845-34-9
ISBN 978-1-891845-34-5

TREATING PEDIATRIC BED-WETTING WITH
ACUPUNCTURE & CHINESE MEDICINE
by Robert Helmer
ISBN 1-891845-33-0
ISBN 978-1-891845-33-8

TREATISE on the SPLEEN & STOMACH: A Translation
and annotation of Li Dong-yuan's Pi Wei Lun
by Bob Flaws
ISBN 0-936185-41-4
ISBN 978-0-936185-41-5

THE TREATMENT OF CARDIOVASCULAR
ISEASES WITH CHINESE MEDICINE
by Simon Becker, Bob Flaws & Robert Casañas, MD
ISBN 1-891845-27-6
ISBN 978-1-891845-27-7

THE TREATMENT OF DIABETES MELLITUS WITH
CHINESE MEDICINE
by Bob Flaws, Lynn Kuchinski & Robert Casañas, M.D.
ISBN 1-891845-21-7
ISBN 978-1-891845-21-5

THE TREATMENT OF DISEASE IN TCM, Vol. 1:
Diseases of the Head & Face, Including Mental &
Emotional Disorders New Edition
by Philippe Sionneau & Lü Gang
ISBN 0-936185-69-4
ISBN 978-0-936185-69-9

THE TREATMENT OF DISEASE IN TCM, Vol. II:
Diseases of the Eyes, Ears, Nose, & Throat
by Sionneau & Lü
ISBN 0-936185-73-2
ISBN 978-0-936185-73-6

THE TREATMENT OF DISEASE IN TCM, Vol. III:
Diseases of the Mouth, Lips, Tongue, Teeth & Gums
by Sionneau & Lü
ISBN 0-936185-79-1
ISBN 978-0-936185-79-8

THE TREATMENT OF DISEASE IN TCM, Vol IV:
Diseases of the Neck, Shoulders, Back, & Limbs
by Phi lippe Sion neau & Lü Gang
ISBN 0-936185-89-9
ISBN 978-0-936185-89-7

THE TREATMENT OF DISEASE IN TCM, Vol V:
Diseases of the Chest & Abdomen
by Philippe Sionneau & Lü Gang
ISBN 1-891845-02-0
ISBN 978-1-891845-02-4

THE TREATMENT OF DISEASE IN TCM, Vol VI:
Diseases of the Urogential System & Proctology
by Phi lippe Sion neau & Lü Gang
ISBN 1-891845-05-5
ISBN 978-1-891845-05-5

THE TREATMENT OF DISEASE IN TCM, Vol VII:
General Symptoms
by Philippe Sion neau & Lü Gang
ISBN 1-891845-14-4
ISBN 978-1-891845-14-7

THE TREATMENT OF EXTERNAL DISEASES WITH
ACUPUNCTURE & MOXIBUSTION
by Yan Cui-lan and Zhu Yun-long, trans. by Yang
Shou-zhong
ISBN 0-936185-80-5
ISBN 978-0-936185-80-4

THE TREATMENT OF MODERN WESTERN
MEDICAL DISEASES WITH CHINESE MEDICINE
by Bob Flaws & Philippe Sionneau
ISBN 1-891845-20-9
ISBN 978-1-891845-20-8

UNDERSTANDING THE DIFFICULT PATIENT: A
Guide for Practitioners of Oriental Medicine
by Nancy Bilello, RN, L.ac.
ISBN 1-891845-32-2
ISBN 978-1-891845-32-1

WESTERN PHYSICAL EXAM SKILLS FOR
PRACTITIONERS OF ASIAN MEDICINE
by Bruce H. Robinson & Honora Lee Wolfe
ISBN 1-891845-48-9
ISBN 978-1-891845-48-2

YI LIN GAI CUO (Correcting the Errors in the Forest
of Medicine)
by Wang Qing-ren
ISBN 1-891845-39-X
ISBN 978-1-891845-39-0

70 ESSENTIAL CHINESE HERBAL FORMULAS
by Bob Flaws
ISBN 0-936185-59-7
ISBN 978-0-936185-59-0

160 ESSENTIAL CHINESE READY-MADE
MEDICINES
by Bob Flaws
ISBN 1-891945-12-8
ISBN 978-1-891945-12-3

630 QUESTIONS & ANSWERS ABOUT CHINESE
HERBAL MEDICINE:
A Work book & Study Guide
by Bob Flaws
ISBN 1-891845-04-7
ISBN 978-1-891845-04-8

260 ESSENTIAL CHINESE MEDICINALS
by Bob Flaws
ISBN 1-891845-03-9
ISBN 978-1-891845-03-1

750 QUESTIONS & ANSWERS ABOUT
ACUPUNCTURE
Exam Preparation & Study Guide
by Fred Jennes
ISBN 1-891845-22-5
ISBN 978-1-891845-22-2